'Should we call the doctor?' is a question every family asks themselves from time to time. Often it causes them unnecessary worry. *The Family Medical Handbook* is designed to advise and reassure. Written by an experienced GP, it clearly explains, in an easily understood A-Z format, whether a disorder can be self-managed, or is more serious, or requires immediate medical attention. The alphabetical entries include, in addition to information on common illness and more serious ailments, advice on many other subjects which relate to family life and the health and well-being of its members. In some general chapters the author provides guidance on a wide range of problems, including the care of old people and the normal development of babies and children. *The Family Medical Handbook* is a dependable reference aid for every home's bookshelf.

The Family Medical Handbook

An A-Z guide

DAVID KELLETT CARDING
MA MB B CHIR

London
UNWIN PAPERBACKS
Boston   Sydney

First published in Great Britain by Pan Books Limited 1970 as
The Home Medical Guide
New edition published by Faber and Faber Limited 1976
Second edition published as *The Family Medical Handbook* 1981
First published in Unwin Paperbacks 1981

This book is copyright under the Berne Convention. All rights are reserved. Apart from any fair dealing for the purpose of private study, research, criticism or review, as permitted under the Copyright Act, 1956, no part of this publication may be reproduced, stored in a retrieval system, or transmitted, in any form or by any means, electronic, electrical chemical, mechanical, optical, photocopying, recording or otherwise, without the prior permission of the copyright owner. Enquiries should be sent to the publishers at the undermentioned address:

UNWIN ® PAPERBACKS
40 Museum Street, London WC1A 1LU

© David Kellett Carding 1981

British Library Cataloguing in Publication Data

Carding, David Kellett
The family medical handbook – 2nd ed.
1. Diseases – Dictionaries
I. Title   II. Home medical guide
616'.003   R121   80-41219

ISBN 0-04-616020-5

Condition of Sale. This book is sold subject to the condition that it shall not, by way of trade or otherwise, be lent, re-sold, hired out or otherwise circulated, without the Publishers' prior consent in any form of binding or cover other than that in which it is published and without a similar condition including this condition being imposed on the purchaser.

Set in 10 on 12pt Bembo by V & M Graphics, Aylesbury, Bucks.,
and printed in Great Britain
by Hunt Barnard Printing Ltd, Aylesbury, Bucks.

RECORD OF VACCINATIONS

NAME _____ | DATES

DATE OF BIRTH _____

SMALL POX

WHOOPING COUGH

DIPHTHERIA

TETANUS

POLIOMYELITIS

MEASLES

GERMAN MEASLES

B.C.G.

OTHERS

to J. K. C.

Acknowledgements

If I had remembered all that I should have learned from patients and colleagues, this would have been a better book.

It is a pleasure to acknowledge the help of Miss P. Downie, F.C.S.P., Editor, Nursing and Medical Books, Faber & Faber, in the preparation of this edition, which continues to enjoy the benefit of Audrey Besterman's illustrations, and to thank Mrs. Joan Harper for research and typing.

I hope that any pharmacist friends who read this will accept my acknowledgement of the wise and patient guidance which I and many other doctors have received from members of their profession.

Introduction

Medical advice is now so readily available in a great part of the United Kingdom that much of what used to appear in books on home treatment is no longer required; but there are many disorders which do not need the attention of a doctor and which, if recognized, will respond to simple treatment and the body's natural powers of recovery. If such cases could be confidently and competently treated at home, family doctors would have more time to spend on patients whom they now have to refer to hospital, and waiting lists would benefit.

This book tries to show what can safely be dealt with at home and what needs medical help. It is written by a family doctor and represents his personal opinions, avoiding controversial matters as far as possible. Some items of general medical information and some notes on preventive medicine have also been included.

In previous editions, I tried to avoid controversial subjects, but some problems now under public discussion require people to make their own decisions, and as a contribution to that process, I have added notes on whooping cough vaccination and home confinements; and two further notes on cot deaths and the use of casualty departments, both of which deserve wider understanding. The main contents are arranged alphabetically, but as childhood, adolescence and old age are periods when advice is most often needed, a general survey of them is given in the first three chapters.

Code letters are printed against some entries as a guide to the need for medical advice. The key to the code is printed overleaf and on the inside back cover of the book. Except where used for emphasis, the printing of a word in *italics* indicates an entry of that title in the Alphabetical Section.

Most doses are given in 5 ml spoonfuls and milligrams (mg), the legal standard since 1969. The 5 ml spoon is about the size of an average teaspoon, and is obtainable from a pharmacist. Domestic measures have been retained in a few situations in which they seem appropriate.

I no longer give prices for books and pamphlets, as the only certain thing is that they will be wrong by the time they are read. Changes of address have caused difficulties; the addresses given were correct when going to press.

● **If the patient is not within the scope of home care, or worsens in spite of it, or if there is any uncertainty, a doctor should be consulted.**

Key

- UU Medical aid necessary without delay.
- U Medical aid necessary within one to three hours, depending on severity and distance from hospital.
- D Ask the doctor to call the same day.
- V Ask the doctor to call the same day (or the day following if the message is sent late).
- S Attend the doctor's next surgery session.
- C Attend the doctor's surgery as soon as convenient.

All treatments suggested are for otherwise healthy persons of average build. Look up in the alphabetical section the name of any remedy suggested before using it.

Anyone who is already under treatment by his doctor should consult him before attempting any but the simplest home treatment.

● **If a patient is not within the scope of home care, or worsens in spite of it, or if there is any uncertainty, a doctor should be consulted.**

'Family Doctor' booklets mentioned in the text are published by the B.M.A., Family Doctor Publications, B.M.A. House, Tavistock Square, London WC1H 9JP, who will send a priced list of publications on receipt of a stamped addressed envelope.

Newborn

Before birth, a baby has food and oxygen piped to it, is kept warm, and protected from injury. After birth it has to learn to breathe, eat, and warm itself, all for the first time, without rehearsal. If it is a first baby, its parents are also learning. It is an anxious time.

There are wide variations in the normal range of food intake, sleep, bowel action, and other activities. This was not always recognized in some of the earlier advice given to mothers, and too rigid insistence on quantities of food, feeding times, sleep requirements, etc, can cause unnecessary anxiety. (*Strength* of the feed is another matter. Accurate measuring is very important.)

As soon as air is taken into the lungs and food into the stomach, the possibility arises that germs or poisons may go the same way. Germs with which an older person has reached a state of armed truce may cause severe infection in an infant if transferred from the throat by talking or coughing, or from the lower bowel by unwashed hands. No one with a cold or cough should enter the baby's room; if the mother catches a cold she should gargle her throat with *isotonic saline*, and put on a gauze or paper mask before tending the baby. Other children should be discouraged from peering into the cot and the kissing of babies should be abandoned, perhaps even by the mother, who can show her love by other forms of caress. Hands should always be washed after using the lavatory, and immediately before preparing a feed in utensils sterilized as the mother will have been shown.

A baby's first efforts at keeping warm may not be sufficient, and it will need help until its 'thermostat' develops. The mother should be sure that she understands the instructions of her midwife or nurse about maintaining her baby's body warmth.

Unless it is known that a baby can breathe almost silently, a parent may lie awake at night fearing that it has stopped breathing. The remedy is to get out of bed as soon as the fear arises and reassure oneself.

At first, a baby's food intake is entirely in fluid form. Nourishment is removed from the feed as it passes through the intestines, and at the far end enough water is extracted to meet the body's fluid requirements. If the feeds are too small, so much water may be extracted that the motions become solid, or hard, small in bulk, and passed infrequently. If the feeding is right, the motion will resemble scrambled eggs, and will usually be passed several times a day, becoming less frequent when the baby is a few weeks old, when there may be an interval of one or two days between stools. Breast-fed babies usually have looser stools, sometimes with mucus (jelly); those of bottle-fed babies are more 'formed' — of a definite shape — with no fluid or mucus.

Diarrhoea is rare in breast-fed babies. Unusually frequent stools may be caused by something laxative finding its way into the milk from the mother's diet — plums, apricots, excessive green vegetables, or vegetable laxatives — and when this is eliminated, the trouble stops. True diarrhoea, with passage of unusually frequent liquid stools, sometimes with mucus or blood, is a sign that infection has entered the system, and help must be asked for (D). Infection may first affect the stomach, causing vomiting, followed by diarrhoea. In either case, while waiting for the doctor, it is important to try to keep up the intake of fluid, because the stomach will be very sensitive and may throw back a full-strength artificial feed as a clotted vomit. Dissolve three level 5ml spoonfuls of glucose or granulated sugar in six ounces (200 ml) of previously boiled water. Calculate three fluid ounces (90 ml) of this mixture for each pound of body weight for the whole day, and give in one- or two-hourly feeds of corresponding size at body temperature. With a smaller intake, the stomach will not send its usual message to the intestines and bowels to move along and make room. The tendency for the bowel to act when a feed is taken is sometimes mistaken for the feed 'going right through him', and feeds are withheld for that reason. This worsens the situation, as it is essential gradually to replace the lost fluid. If this is not done, the baby becomes 'dehydrated', stops passing urine, becomes listless, with sunken eyes and the patch of soft skin on top of its head sinking below the level of the scalp. This is serious and calls for early help (**U**).

'Possetting' is a harmless condition in which a little of the feed is returned as a creamy or clotted fluid when the baby is laid down. This serves as a reminder that the baby should never have a pillow, but should lie on a firm mattress whose cover is tightly stretched and cannot ruck or form pockets, in which vomit might collect and obstruct breathing if the child should turn into it.

The old saying is 'a possetting baby thrives'. If a baby who returns its feed does not thrive, it may be suffering from the rarer condition of rumination. In this, the baby forms the habit if regurgitating its feed (often a sweet artificial feed) over and over again into its mouth, apparently because it likes the taste of it. At each return, some feed spills from the mouth, and gives rise to the typical picture of an ailing child whose pillow is constantly wet with regurgitated feed. Medical advice is needed (**C**) and the condition usually responds quickly to reorganization of the feed.

Another unusual condition is projectile vomiting — a literal description, for the vomit, occuring shortly after a feed, is shot several feet across the room. It is caused by pyloric stenosis — narrowing of the outlet from the stomach — and is treated medically or surgically according to its severity. A less dramatic projectile vomit is sometimes caused by hiatus hernia (described under *Heartburn*). The doctor should be consulted as soon as the condition is recognized — (**C** or **V** according to severity).

The word 'wind' is much heard during the first months of childhood. It is part of the routine of feeding to 'get the wind up' after each meal: that is, to allow the escape from the stomach of air which has been sucked in with the feed and swallowed.

The baby is sat on his mother's knee and bent forward a little over his own left knee. From time to time he can be lifted under his armpits and allowed to dangle for a few seconds, or be held on his mother's chest, looking over her shoulder. In the course of 15 or 20 minutes (often less, occasionally more) he will give one or two good belches, and can then be put down. Some babies seem to manage better if a short break is made in mid-feed for de-winding.

Some bottle-fed babies do not 'go down' comfortably after their feed. This can be caused by a feed which is too weak, too cool, or too difficult to get — the teat having too small a hole. The latter is easily remedied with a red-hot needle. When the feed is made, it should run freely from the teat on tilting the bottle, and should feel comfortably warm on the back of the hand. The proportions and sweetness of the feed should be advised by the doctor or clinic; as a rough guide to quantity, it can be taken that unless a baby is having at least 2½ fluid ounces (75 ml) of liquid intake for each pound of its weight in 24 hours, it is going short.

A baby who cries, getting red in the face and pulling up his legs, is sometimes said to have 'the wind'. What it does have is pain somewhere, not necessarily in the abdomen, and not necessarily due to windy colic. If it continues for more than an hour or two, or returns later, medical advice should be sought (**S** or **D** according to severity). There is an odd condition, cause unknown, called 'evening' colic. The baby cries at a regular time each evening. It seldom continues after the age of four months, and most cases are relieved by medical treatment (**C**).

Constipation in babies is usually due to insufficient fluid intake. Once this is adjusted, the trouble usually disappears, but it may call for 'Milk of Magnesia' in a *total daily dose of half to one 5 ml spoonful,* divided into 2 or 3 small doses, for a short time.

Older relatives, who recall starting mixed feeding at 7 or 8 months, may be surprised how early it is now advised. Many experts believe that mixed feeding is sometimes being attempted too early — particularly the introduction of wheat products — and current advice is that four months is the earliest at which mixed feeding should be started, that the dried milk and sugar content of artificial feeds should never be increased above that advised by doctor, nurse or health visitor, and that *no salt* should be added either to feeds or to mixed feeds, unless advised.

Little mention has been made above of difficulties with breast-fed babies. They happen much less often, as might be expected, for breast milk is the designed product, and is usually superior to all substitutes. So much so, that it is worth making an effort to overcome the initial practical, and subsequent social, difficulties, in order to continue breast feeding whenever it is possible.

If infection makes its way into the breathing system (usually by contact with a common cold), the most frequently affected site will be the nose, with snuffling and obstructed breathing, leading to difficulty in sucking the feed. This last may be met by giving smaller quantities more often, stopping frequently to allow mouth breathing. The nostrils may be cleared occasionally using small twists of cotton wool, very gently. The cot may be tilted some three or four inches to raise the baby's head (never use a pillow), and a few drops of eucalyptus oil on a handkerchief fastened at waist level below the outer clothes, so that the vapour rises to his nose without risk of the oil getting into his eyes. Should infection spread to the ear the baby may be restless, often feverish, and cry from pain; a different cry from that which a baby may make at a regular interval before its next feed is due (**S** or **D**). It can come on at any time, or be continuous, is more intense and often higher pitched, and may prevent feeding rather than be stopped by it. A similar situation may accompany an inflamed throat, though pain is less prominent and unwillingness to swallow more so (**S**, **D**, or **V**). Note that ear inflammation may give rise to vomiting or diarrhoea without the baby being obviously in pain — the condition will be found by the doctor investigating the case. A baby with a *cough* should be seen by a doctor (**S** or **D**). Most of them will have easily recoverable tracheitis, but some may have bronchitis and some pneumonia or bronchiolitis or asthmatic bronchitis (**U** or **D** according to severity). In pneumonia, a cough may not be very obvious, but the baby breathes rapidly, is feverish and ill and the nostrils may dilate as he breathes. In bronchiolitis and asthmatic bronchitis there is added wheezing as the child breathes out.

If unfit to be taken to the doctor, the baby is kept in a warmed room until he comes, with the cot tilted as described above. The air should be kept moist by having a large bowl (or baby's bath) of water on the floor near the source of heat; or, if breathing is difficult, in a steam-filled room, as described under *cough*.

Often a baby who is ill cannot regulate his body temperature. It should not lie out of doors or in a cold room, but should be kept in a warm moist air. It should be well wrapped, but a hot water bottle is best avoided except on medical advice.

During the first year it is advisable to protect a baby by vaccination against whooping cough, diphtheria, tetanus (lockjaw), and poliomyelitis (see *Vaccination*). Vaccination against measles is usually given in the second year. Smallpox vaccination is now only given in the U.K. if the child is going to a smallpox area. This may be the place to remind mothers of a rather frequent lapse in infant management. Surprisingly often, a mother, partly through nervousness and partly from a wish to 'play down' what is being done, laughs when an injection is given. It is better to gather the baby to her and quietly comfort him. The next visit to a surgery or clinic may then bring a memory of maternal care rather than of pain.

When a baby is the family favourite, other children may try to please him with offers of painted toys or furniture — beware lest the paint contain lead. (If bought as children's toys, the seller will usually be able to assure you about this.) Another favourite offering is the coloured iron tablets which many mothers need during and after a pregnancy. These can be fatal if eaten by babies and young children, and if any are found to have been taken, immediate help at hospital or from the doctor is essential (UU.).

Teeth usually begin to appear between the 5th and 10th month. An account of *teething* will be found in the Alphabetical

Section. Consult also *Deafness in children* and *Squint* for the early recognition and treatment of these.

A baby can't move but sunlight does. Make sure that the sun will not climb out of the shade in which you have left the baby, and burn him.

From the Second Year to Adolescence

When a child does become mobile, a complete overhaul of the home arrangements is needed. He will be filled with an urge to explore and investigate; to climb on stools and pull saucepan handles, poke hair grips into electric sockets, switch bedside lamps with wet fingers, or unscrew their fittings. Everything liftable will be picked up and tested in the mouth to decide if it should be eaten. The only way to achieve even moderate peace of mind is to take each room in turn and spend time working out how every article and fitting can be dangerous. Extend the exercise to passages, doors, garden, garage, and car; arrange a properly secure cupboard for medicines, including familiar home remedies, especially aspirin, paracetamol, and iron tablets, and another for poisons. In a home in which children have not lived before, the list of dangers can be hair-raising, and the RoSPA pamphlet mentioned on page 17 should help.

This is a time when an experienced and tactful grandmother is beyond price. Failing such good fortune, recourse must be had to one of the publications designed to guide parents; always remembering that few children are 'typical' or 'average' all through, and that an author cannot describe the whole range of childhood's differences without losing the value of his book as a general guide.

During the first year the baby will have been vaccinated against diphtheria, tetanus (lockjaw), probably whooping cough, and poliomyelitis. Measles vaccination is given in the second year, and the entry *Vaccination* in the Alphabetical Section should be consulted for guidance. It is wise to keep a written record of vaccinations (see page v), and of any illnesses, with dates.

Most children start to walk between the ages of 12 and 18 months. Some who do not are simply late developers, but a proportion have some disability, and the doctor's advice should be sought if walking is delayed after 18 months. Soon after he starts to walk, a child may be seen to be limping, or his back may seem bent to one side (the latter may be noticed much earlier, during the first few months). If brought to medical notice early, some cases of hip and spinal trouble can be spotted in time for treatment to be effective. At this stage, it may be feared that a child is bow-legged. What is usually noticed is the natural curve of the shin bone which becomes less obvious as growth proceeds, as also does the tendency to 'toe-in' when walking. Bowing of the whole leg, including the knee joint, is rare and if found needs medical advice.

There is a wide variation in the development of speech. Broadly, most babies say 'Dada', 'Mama', 'Ta', or variants of these, at 12 months. At 15 months, some words are clearly spoken, and short 2 or 3 word sentences ('Peter wants drink') at 2 years.

Teething is usually completed during the third year, and the eruption of the last four molars may give rise to ill temper lasting several days. If the cause is recognized, it is reasonable to treat the discomfort with half an *aspirin* tablet (or 2 children's aspirins) morning and evening. The child may go off food at this time, and if the physical cause is unrecognized, the foundation of future trouble can be laid. Emerging independence of spirit may already have led to refusal of food, particularly if this is found to produce a gratifying increase in parental attention, and a mistaken effort to force feeding which produces pain can result in a damaged relationship which takes time to heal. The food should be offered as usual, and if not eaten should be removed after the time usually taken for a meal. Comment should be neutral and minimal — 'sorry you don't feel hungry'. Dispose of the food, and of the temptation to serve it for the next meal, which should be prepared as usual and dealt with in the same way if rejected. If sore gums were responsible, the appetite will return in a few days, and feeding will be resumed, unless a manipulative mood has developed on finding that more attention is gained by refusing food than by eating it. If that has been allowed to happen, it is important that no emotional reaction should be shown, but opportunity may be taken to cancel or refuse some outing or treat, with the sorrowful explanation that 'I'm afraid it would tire you too much, as you haven't had enough to eat today'.

A child can manage quite well without food for several days, provided he drinks the usual amount, and drinks *in his own mug* should be left where he can take them without arousing comment. If the situation is felt to be out of control, consult your doctor before physical signs of malnutrition appear. Try to see him alone first, to give a short account of the situation. It is heartbreaking to watch an astute toddler rejoicing in his parents' account of the situation into which they have got themselves.

Another cause of temporary refusal of food is an inflamed throat, and observation may show that the act of swallowing is painful. The *temperature* may be found to be raised (S, V, or D, according to severity).

Delay in reading and writing gives rise to justifiable anxiety. Its causes range from late development (which is self-correcting) to constitutional difficulty in remembering the shapes of letters or the sounds of words. Between these lie a range of difficulties related to emotional strains, whose effect can be worsened by mismanagement of such things as lefthandedness, deafness, or short sight. Recognition of the cause may need specialized experience, and any child whose reading or writing ability is considerably lower than others of his age should be investigated. In larger cities, the school authorities have arrangements for this. In smaller communities the matter should be taken up with the education authority, in consultation with the school staff. Many cases will respond to an alteration in management, and 'parent counselling' plays an important part. In others, this will have to be reinforced by special training. Parents can be reassured that constitutional reading/writing difficulty (dyslexia) does not go hand-in-hand with mental backwardness, and that it can affect children of all grades of intelligence (see British Dyslexia Association, p. 264).

Unrecognized *deafness in children* can give rise to a suspicion of *backwardness*. See the relevant entries.

Two causes of anxiety for those starting their first parenthood are inability to judge the seriousness of early physical illness, and fear that they may unwittingly mismanage their child's development. For the first, the commoner symptoms and illnesses of children are described in the Alphabetical Section of this book. Remember that the doctor/patient relationship will survive more unnecessary calls requested early in the day, than it will necessary ones left until late. . .

The first approaches to child management may be helped by a short account of the general climate of childhood and of some of the miscalculations which well-intentioned parents can make. What follows represents the view of one family doctor about a controversial subject, and should be taken as such.

Until the age of 5 or 6, a child's thoughts are chiefly concerned with his own inner feelings, and though the outside world is increasingly explored, impressions of it are knit into internal patterns of thought and imagination, rather than appreciated as facts. In the seventh year, interest turns outwards to observe objects, facts, and situations as they are, rather than as things to think about, and to participate in them consciously, as outside happenings. In boys, this period is marked by the development of aggressiveness, a normal feature between the ages of 7 and 13 years.

At puberty, the mind turns in on itself again to battle through the confusions of adolescence, and that, above all, is the time when the foundations laid in the first years are tested.

The ideal childhood is spent in communion with both parents and other members of the family. A child is handicapped to the extent that this is deficient, though the degree of handicap will depend on his own strength of character and the conditions in which he grows up. No theoretical learning can compensate for the lack of a simple code of conduct on which actions and decisions can be seen to be based, or of the constant, outgoing and tranquil expression of parental love.

In early life, children are strongly attached emotionally to their mother, and for this reason she should avoid working away from home unless it is economically necessary. The fact that the father's chief role is to support and help the mother at this time can obscure the need for him to establish and keep a close relationship with his child. A common and harmful situation is that in which a father devotes so much energy to developing his career that he has little left for family relationships; the extent of his daily fatigue persuading him that in making good provision for his family he has done his share, and that the care of home and children justly falls to his wife. However well he may convince himself, it is a hard fact that the emotional demands of childhood need to be supplied by both mother and father in different ways, and a father should not only be providing for and protecting his family, but should be felt to be doing so by every member of it. A situation which prevents that happening should be closely examined with a view to alteration, either of it or of his attitude to it. Fathers should also beware of the 'stiff upper lip' attitude towards male relationships once prevalent. If this leads to the rejection of gestures of affection from a young son, it can have a delayed effect in prolonging the short homosexual phase through which most children pass after puberty, as a boy reaches for the male affection previously denied him. It need not be feared that responsiveness will lead to undesirable softness. A father who is, in the current phrase, 'involved' with his son is in a far better position to breed courage in him than one who stands on the side-lines calling for valour.

If the lack of attention is a father's commonest parental mistake, it may be that excess of it is a mother's, although this is not an exclusively maternal fault! Exaggeration of the maternal instinct to protect and comfort the child can lead to its being shielded from any encounter with adversity; too many treats are given, not for the child's pleasure, but in the hope of evoking a response pleasurable to the parent. A similar attempt to produce a response from a child (who by that time wants only to be left in peace for a while) leads to 'building up' everything that is going to happen, so that when it does happen the reality disappoints expectation. The result can be a spoiled child believing that the world exists for his pleasure, and reacting to any mishap as he did to the first unpleasant thing that ever happened to him — by crying.

Delicate judgement is needed to bring home the existence of harmful and evil things to a two-year-old, but he needs gradually to be brought to understand that some things are bad and can hurt him and that his actions or omissions can hurt or help others. He must always know that he can count on the support and patience of each parent in encountering and mastering bad situations.

In the second and third years a child will increasingly need direction in managing his widening contacts, especially when the emergence of self-will in the third year takes over from the exploratory drive of the second. It is important that this direction be firmly based, explainable, and explained. Disobedience of an unthinking instruction which could not be justified in level argument puts the parent in a difficult position. The alternatives are to withdraw gracefully ('I'm sorry, I made a mistake. I should have said—'), to emit a smokescreen of justification which may be expected but not believed, or to punish because, right or wrong, one has not been obeyed. The last is not now considered a sound basis for child management, although in an imperfect world 'because I say so' must occasionally be the ultimate argument.

Frustration, fatigue, and the need for a few minutes' quiet, probably cause most of the the hurried decisions which are later regretted. Few children grasp readily the idea that an adult can become tired, and none will believe it of an autocratic parent who enforces discipline by giving unexplained orders. One who gives decisions after reflection, deals firmly with questions arising, and is not afraid to say she doesn't know, is in a better position. She will already have shown that she is not infallible and can, without loss of prestige, say that she is tired, and needs to be left sitting quietly alone for as long as it takes for a favourite record to be played. (Don't say 'for ten minutes'. You will say it as if it were a short time, but to a child ten minutes is an interminable wait.) The problem of how to deal with disobedience of a reasonable order depends partly on how far the disobedience can be shown to have had bad results. A painful minor injury will probably do all that is needed towards avoidance of its cause in future; but for some things such as straying in the road or meddling with electricity, one disobedience is one too many, and if serious consequences are escaped, punishment should follow. The non-violent will immediately, levelly, and sorrowfully pronounce sentence of deprivation of some treat or favourite pursuit within the next few hours; don't drag it on, and *never* 'wait till your father gets home.'* Others will unhurriedly administer two or three firm spanks without displaying emotion. Suppress the natural impulse to give a good shake or a wild swipe in the first flush of anxiety produced by the event.

Inquisitiveness is natural to the human race, and precautions are needed against the possible harmful results of exploratory urges — as far as possible by making safe, rather than by forbidding. If the answer to a question is known, give it; if not, say so and try to find it. It is useful to have a single volume encyclopedia which can be consulted quickly, and which children will later be encouraged to use.

The readier one is to answer questions, the less likely one is to form the habit of turning them aside; an advantage when the time comes to acquaint a child with knowledge of reproduction. Indeed, a time for formal initiation need never come if questions are answered when asked, simply and without embarrassment. Quite young children can be told that babies

---

* This refers to toddlers. Older boys in the aggressive phase already discussed cannot always be handled by a woman, and the father should make it understood that anything done in his absence which would not have been done in his presence must be accounted for as soon as it comes to his notice. The mother's task is to deal with any occurrence unemotionally, and to report it promptly and without exaggeration as soon as her husband has had time to cast off the cares of the day. The position of a widow at this stage of a son's life is particularly difficult. Help may be gained by membership of a club (such as a Cruse Club, 126 Sheen Road, Richmond, Surrey TW9 1UR, for widows, and Gingerbread or one of its local groups — write to 35 Wellington Street, London WC2 — for one-parent families).

grow in mummy's tummy, and that daddy helps by giving mummy the seed for the baby and by looking after her while the baby is growing. Later, the mechanics can be explained by demonstrating the sex organs of pets and explaining that the seed is made in the testicles, and given to the female through the penis. There is much to be said for ensuring that a child has a knowledge of reproduction before puberty, so that it forms part of his general store of knowledge when he enters that disturbing phase.

The emerging adolescent may at any time need unobtrusive support, more by hint or example than by direct interference, and the more vigilant a parent is for the early signs of trouble, the sooner he may be able to adjust the balance of stresses responsible. Direct advice should be given sparingly, after reflection and as between equals; suggestion more often, and a direct order rarely.

On reaching the borders of adolescence, after a childhood spent in the constructive atmosphere suggested, a child may still have to contend with hazards, as the surge of mental energy turns inward to a mind not yet able to form a balanced view of his place in the home, the school, and the world. This flow of energy turns most readily into the developing channels of sexual interest, and in excess may be more troublesome to boys than to girls, in so far as the male function is the more aggressive and exploratory. A child who has been able to master a hobby or activity is usually better able to keep in balance, and it can be wondered how far failure to muster concentration and application for this is due to constitutional difference, and how far it may result from lack of adult interest.

The adolescent 'drifter' seems to live a more stressful life than his more phlegmatic and methodical companions, perhaps because almost every activity involves an encounter with the unknown, unrelated to any systematic programme or regular occupation; and such young people need the anchorage of parental interest and of predictable parental behaviour, although natural rebelliousness may lead them to scoff at it. In them, the occasional occurrence of mental illness can be more difficult to recognize and more easily mistaken for indolence or wilfulness. Most doctors are accustomed to supervise more or less anxiously a handful of young people passing through varying degrees of mental disorder. In neurosis and depression, the symptoms vary from procrastination, restlessness, indecision, and loss of application to the abandonment of all intellectual effort and deep melancholy. *Schizophrenia* may at first be indistinguishable from the vagaries of adolescence, with increasing churlishness, loss of initiative and emotional response, and increasing personal untidiness. Any behaviour which seems to lie outside the range of variation normal to that person, and particularly any sudden worsening of the mood or behaviour, should alert the family to the possibility of mental illness, and medical advice should be sought, preferably by means of an interview with the doctor before the patient sees him. It does seem that more of the excesses of youth than have been recognized may be due to temporary mental illness and may be amenable to treatment.

Dissatisfaction with the state of the world and exasperation with the generation thought to be responsible for it are normal (and on balance beneficial) qualities of adolescence. Parents who have throughout encouraged an open, speculative, and liberal attitude will not find it difficult to meet this situation and to lead towards avenues of social responsibility. On the other hand, it is now that the authoritarian may reap the whirlwind when he feels the full force of the adolescent's resentment.

It will be seen that, in so far as it is attainable by human effort, a tranquil adolescence resembles a good asparagus bed. Work should have started long before.

Further Reading. When I wrote the original version of this section, I had not read the masterly final chapter of the late Dr J.D. Hadfield's *Childhood and Adolescence*. First published in 1962, it was reprinted in 1974 in a Pelican edition. I do hope it stays in print.

Babies and Toddlers
Understanding your Child (Birth to 5 years)
So Now You Know About Sex (for 12 years upwards)
These are all Family Doctor Publications

Safe as Houses (Accident Prevention) Pamphlet HS 139, and *First Steps to Safety*, both obtainable from RoSPA, Cannon House, Priory Queensway, Birmingham B1 6BS

Alone Again. Help for the divorced, separated and bereaved. By Angela Willans and obtainable from the National Marriage Guidance Council, Herbert Gray College, Little Church Street, Rugby

Old Age

We have to deal not so much with age, as the effects of ageing. These can be crippling in a man of 65 or negligible in one of 80. Whenever degeneration of brain or body begins to affect function, then the victim and those about him are confronting senility, and it must be decided if he or she can continue life as before, or will need help and supervision. The problem is usually encountered when it affects one or both parents, or an aunt or uncle to whom one is next of kin; and the circumstances vary widely.

The first need is for as accurate a picture as possible of the state of affairs. For this, one should consult the patient's doctor, and he will feel more free if he knows the approach is being made with the patient's knowledge and approval — indeed, in most circumstances it will be impossible for him to discuss the case without them.

The doctor will be able to describe the patient's disability, and usually to give an idea of what may be expected in the way of recovery or worsening; and of the time scale involved, though the more experienced he is, the less he will be likely to commit himself — particularly on expectation of life. He will advise on the likelihood of the patient continuing to live alone, cook for and care for himself; the risks of falling, of heart attacks, or the momentary fits of unconsciousness to which many are prone, and in which they may injure themselves.

When the effects of senility first appear, it may be found that they can be eased by a number of medical and domestic measures, which have not until then appeared necessary. Medically the doctor may be able to arrange for rehabilitation of weakened limbs, treatment to strengthen a failing heart, to correct minor anaemia or malnutrition, and help failing hearing and eyesight. The dentist should be asked to protect the patient's weakened digestive powers by providing false teeth, if needed, or to ensure that those he has fit properly. (Advice on the possibility of financial help with this may be had from Social Security offices.) In these and other directions a number of small advantages may be gained which lead to an overall improvement in health.

Attendance may be possible at an old people's clinic each week for chiropody, simple physiotherapy, rehabilitation of balance, comradeship, and the recognition of minor ailments which the patient would not have thought merited his doctor's attention. When resources are dwindling, every effort should be made to screw the last ounce of efficiency out of what remains, so that a small reserve can be established. This calls for a great expenditure of time, skill, and ingenuity by doctors, social workers, and local authorities; and it would be foolish to pretend that the undermanned and overworked Health and Social Services can always find it. However, a start has been made, and in some places the devotion of individuals is achieving what the community cannot yet provide.

When a small credit balance has been gained, it can be increased by reducing the calls on the patient's strength, some of which will be found to have been wastefully unnecessary. 'Streamlining' the home involves studying every activity the occupant performs, and planning to reduce the energy expended on it. The greatest saving can usually be made in stair climbing. A person weighing eight stone is lifting a hundredweight up ten feet every time she climbs the stairs. Bringing the bed downstairs will abolish that exertion, provided toilet arrangements exist, or can be contrived, on the ground floor. The pleasure of tending a coal fire and the carrying of coals in and ashes out should be sacrificed in favour of electric, gas, or oil heating, and electric switches and gas taps should be of the latest safety design. Attention is given to the lighting of any dark passages, raised thresholds are either painted a contrasting colour or fitted with ramps, and a handrail put along the wall. Loose rugs should be replaced by overall carpeting — not necessarily 'fitted' — a haircord square often fits comfortably and can be turned from time to time to equalize wear. Bath mats are abolished, and handrails fitted to help in entering and leaving the bath. A transverse seat hung from the sides of the bath is often needed, and a rubber mat fixing to the *inside* of the bath with suckers can be bought. It prevents the frequent accident caused by a foot slipping while getting out. A common cause of dizziness and fainting is reduced blood flow to the head and brain when the neck is stretched backwards. To avoid this happening, all shelves, fastenings, hooks, clothes airers, etc, should be kept at or below the patient's eye level. Some of these alterations can be carried out by the Social Services Department. The Social Security Office will advise about possible entitlement to supplementary, attendance and disability allowances.

The main meal should be at midday, provided if possible by the Meals on Wheels Service, and the kitchen crockery and apparatus should be reduced to a minimum. It should include an easily-filled vacuum flask in which a hot drink can be kept ready for the morning, having been prepared at the same time as supper. Most older people manage to give themselves a well-balanced diet until they are in the early or middle seventies. After that, they may become forgetful or careless, and their diet deficient, particularly in calcium, vitamins D, B, and C, and protein. Milk and cheese, butter, eggs, meat, liver, peas, leaf vegetables and fresh fruit, tomatoes and yeast preparations will give a good intake of these, but bread, cakes, and jam do not. This is not just a piece of theory. The deficiencies mentioned can, and do, give rise to definite diseases, confusion, and self neglect; and old people, or old couples living alone, fall victims when they can no longer face going out to shop, relying on what can be bought at the door.

If the Meals on Wheels Service can supply five meals a week, these will usually take care of the main nutritional requirements, except for vitamin C, some of which is lost when food has to be stored hot. Fresh vegetables and fruit, especially oranges, will provide it, and can usefully be brought as presents by visitors, who should also try to steal a look at the larder, to make sure that a suitable mixed diet is being taken. This is more important if Meals on Wheels is supplying less than five meals a week. When visiting, one should also check that the home is being kept warm enough. Old people are inactive, have often lost some of their protective fat, and are more susceptible to chilling. It may be a delicate matter to

Old Age 21

suggest that more heat is needed, particularly if money is tight; but it is important, and perhaps a hint could be given to the Old People's Welfare Visiting Committee, or the district nurse or health visitor, if in attendance. Any of these may be in a better position than a relative or friend to take the matter up.

A number of people can be called on for advice and assistance:

1 Social Worker from Local Authority Social Services Department.
2 Health Visitor and Chiropodist from N.H.S. Clinic, Doctor, or Health Centre.
3 District Nurse, through one's own Doctor.
4 Home Help from Local Authority Social Services Department.
5 Meals on Wheels, usually run by the WRVS, reached through the Citizen's Advice Bureau, or the Town Hall.
6 Old People's Welfare Committee. In addition to giving general information about what local facilities are available, a member of the visiting committee can call regularly, both to keep an eye on the patient, and for human contact.
7 Inquiry will often show that children from a local school, Scouts or Guides, are volunteer shoppers for old people.
8 Financial help, or advice on such matters as the cost of staying in an old people's home, its effect on retirement pension, etc, can be had from the local office of the Department of Social Security.
9 Some Local Authorities — usually those in large centres — have laundry facilities for old people.

It is surprising how often the first news of illness comes when a neighbour notices that the milk has not been taken in. Every effort should be made to arrange that either a neighbour or a relative on his way to work calls in each morning for a few minutes. (Remember that the neighbour may herself be old and need support. Her help should not be taken for granted.) Sometimes an alarm system can be arranged with the house next door, and if the window fronts on the road, a red flashing torch light should be provided with which to signal if in trouble at night. In addition to malnutrition, physical illness may upset the mental balance of an old person, leading to confusion or *depression*; and this can also result from isolation (either true remoteness of habitation, or loneliness from insufficient human contact), and desolation, as from the loss of a near relative by death or emigration.

If the patient's disability increases, or if she is obviously not going to be able to live alone, the following alternatives arise:

1 She may be so ill that she has to be admitted to one of the scarce hospital beds as a long-stay patient.
2 Her disability may demand such treatment, but no bed may be available. The long period on the waiting list has then to be passed, either in the home of a relative, or her own home, with such help as can be arranged from doctor, district nurse, Social Services, Meals on Wheels, and volunteer visitors.
3 She may not need hospital care, and could manage well in a sheltered dwelling or Local Authority Home. Application is made through the local Housing Office, or Local Authority Social Services department respectively, and it may be found that a wait of 6 to 24 months is involved. *Put her name on the waiting list now.* A similar wait is usual before admission to a home run by a voluntary society, or the Old People's Welfare Committee. In these, part of the expense is sometimes borne by the Social Services department.
4 If the patient or her relatives can afford the fees, a place can often be found in a nursing home or private old people's home in a matter of a few weeks or months.
5 If all else fails, and the prospect of leaving a near relative alone cannot be faced, space will be found in one's own home, and that is what usually happens.

For whatever reason it has been undertaken, it is a sad fact that the continued success of a home-sharing arrangement usually depends on *maximum separation of the generations*. To the extent that this is not done, conflict and stress are to be expected, and it is best to face the possible embarassment of explaining the

Old Age

arrangements fully at the beginning. Ideally, the old person should have a bed-sitting room containing a washbasin, near to the bathroom and lavatory. (If this is impossible, it is worth considering the use of one of the improved chemical closets now made for campers). If it can be at the end of a passage, so much the better. The floor should be carpeted (no loose mats), the fire efficiently guarded, and there should be a bell by the bedside.

If the occupant is capable, and wishes to cook for herself, one of the smallest electric or gas cookers, and means of boiling a kettle and washing up can be installed. She should not be discouraged from doing her own shopping unless physically unfit, or the weather hazardous. Visits should be 'little and often'. If meals have to be taken in, they serve to punctuate the day, but at such times there will be other things waiting to be done, and it is better to set aside ten minutes mid-morning and afternoon for 'elevenses' and a cup of tea. The old person's room is his or her *home* and should be treated as such, with knocking on the door, 'may I come in?' etc. Children should be encouraged to call as they would if their grandparent were living in another street. They should only stay five or ten minutes — not long enough to exhaust the patience of either party. Once or twice a week, the old person is invited to a meal or to spend the evening; experience will show how often such invitations should be given and returned.

All this may appear cold-blooded, but in the writer's experience, it is the best arrangement for all but the most exceptionally well integrated families. It avoids the growing intolerance and exasperation which easily arise when different generations are brought into too close contact, and allows the development of affection and respect between the older person and different members of the family.

Once a relative has been installed in an old people's home, it is important to keep up family connections and friendships. Avoid the mistake of visiting often at first, afterwards lapsing. Of course, frequent visits are valuable in the first few weeks, while the newcomer is establishing herself. After that, she should be told that she will be visited regularly — eg, on the first Tuesday of each month. From the beginning, quote a time interval that can be observed without fail, for visits are looked forward to eagerly, and disappointment can be intense. Such visiting usually falls on those who are closest, in one sense or another, but they should try to organize visits at longer intervals by more distant relatives. If the inmate is fit for it, an occasional day visit to a relative's or friend's home is worth far more than any trouble taken to arrange it.

(See in the Alphabetical Section for particular troubles which may affect the elderly — eg, *Constipation*.)

There is a full description of special services for the elderly in Phyllis Willmott's *Consumer's Guide to the British Social Services* (Pelican) and the Consumers' Association publish *Health for Old Age* from their Publications Dept., 14 Buckingham St, London, WC2N 6DS

● **If a patient is not within the scope of home care, or worsens in spite of it, or if there is any uncertainty, a doctor should be consulted.**

Topical Subjects under Public Discussion

As I mentioned earlier, I am using a few pages to write notes on some subjects which, at the time of going to press are under public discussion, not all of it equally illuminating. I think some of the difficulties arise when proposals based on technical advances do not take their emotional consequences into account; and this in turn causes diffuse emotional reactions in which the practical advantages of the proposals are forgotten.

Home Confinements. Something of that sort is affecting the present discussions about home confinements. The facts are simple: nearly every pregnancy and confinement are normal and uncomplicated. Good pre-natal care will discover most of the cases which may not be straightforward, and allow special arrangements to be made for them. Of the mothers whose pregnancies pass normally, a small fraction develop unforeseen trouble once they are in labour. If they are being delivered in a fully-staffed hospital, these unforeseeable troubles are recognized and dealt with by specialized staff, using equipment and special experience not available to the midwife and doctor conducting a delivery in the patient's home. So, some lives are saved in hospitals which would have been hazarded at home.

To secure this advantage, a great many mothers are delivered in hospital who, with hindsight, could safely have been confined at home, and among them are some who contrast the degree of personal and emotional satisfaction they enjoyed, with that of a home confinement, to the advantage of the latter.

At this stage, emotion threatens to obscure fact. The fact is that a small number of home confinements will, unpredictably, run into difficulties which could be overcome with the resources of a hospital maternity department, but which might, in home conditions, prove insuperable. The complete technical answer is to conduct all labours in hospital. The more technically advanced the hospital, the less homely it is, and the more a patient misses her home surroundings, human and material. This emotional deficit can be, and usually is, met by the imagination, skill and understanding of the staff, if the country provides money to employ enough of them, which it does not; and if one does not encounter someone whose professional skills have been gained at the expense of human understanding and compassion. This is not unknown.

The workload of a maternity department is unpredictable, both in numbers and difficulty, and there are times when the priority of a safe outcome for mother and baby forces the emotional implications of what is going on into second place, or no place at all, while everybody exerts their skills. The impact of such unadorned technical triumphs depends on the patient. Some with a robust view of childbirth may regard them as part and parcel of a poorly designed arrangement for reproduction, from whose obvious mechanical defects one should remove oneself as soon as is practicable; but if a deep, sometimes mystical, commitment to motherhood includes not only the delights of conception, but also the subsequent pregnancy and delivery, in an act of cosmic participation, the emotional requirements are much more important to the mother.

Many, many mothers have had a complete and satisfying experience from a hospital confinement; I have been able to share in some of them. I have also been present when the insensitivity of one member of the team has made for an imperfect experience; and it is easy to understand anyone who has had, or known of, such, wishing to be delivered at home, close to her family, by professionals whom she knows.

What are the difficulties in arranging a home confinement? They are of various kinds. Assuming from the start that full pre-natal supervision is achieved, and unsuitable cases identified and transferred to specialist care, the next question is whether the house is suitable, for what is, remember, an operation requiring sterility. For good reasons, we no longer perform appendicectomies on people's kitchen tables, and some of these reasons apply to the conduct of labour in a bedroom. If the requirements can be met, who is going to conduct the labour? This needs a trained midwife, supported by a family doctor with special midwifery experience, both of whom will have regularly supervised the pregnancy. Can they be provided? Not everywhere, not only from lack of finances, but because there are not enough midwives to go round. The family doctor 'coyer' is not easy either. He will already be responsible for the care of two or three thousand people, and will usually have arrangements for an off-duty rota to give himself some free time. He may be able to arrange for someone with obstetric experience to deputize for him. If not, he will have to be available for about three weeks around the time of expected delivery, not leaving the neighbourhood. This would be tolerable two or three times a year, but in order to retain his place on the Obstetric List, the doctor would need to be present at, or to conduct twelve or more deliveries a year; that is to say, he must expect to be 'on call' and unable to relax for more than half the year. There are many doctors committed to midwifery who are willing to do this, at whatever cost to their family and social life; but it is not a service which can be demanded as a right, nor one which could be bought or rewarded by any monetary fee likely to be made available.

If one is fortunate in one's professional arrangements, one has still not disposed of the difficulty that a small number of home confinements may develop unexpected and unforeseeable complications when labour is proceeding. It seems inevitable that anyone opting for home confinement must accept this risk, however small it is, and should be willing in advance to exonerate their doctor and midwife from blame for any mishap attributable to their choice. In practice, it is advised that mother and father should sign a written request for the labour to be conducted at home, and an acknowledgement that the doctor has explained the possible disadvantages.

That might be thought to have covered any legal difficulties; but there are more. The law in England now allows a child, upon coming of age, to sue for damages recevied during infancy or before birth, and I am told that, whatever undertaking the parents may give, a doctor or his estate could still be proceeded against for a handicap received at birth, which might have been avoided if delivery had been in hospital. These points are based on legal opinion at national level arising from an enquiry which I made not long ago, and I wonder if those parents and professionals now pressing for more home confinements are aware of them; and if they are, what safeguards they propose.

My own opinion (which takes no account of the variable availability of staff and hospital facilities) is that the present is not the time for a resurgence in home confinements, which should await the solution of the problem of unforeseeable perinatal death and injury. It is sometimes said that we should be looking at the experience of some European countries, where figures are better, although home confinements are frequent. Unfortunately, the latest information reveals an increase in hospital confinements there, for the reasons I have already discussed; and it may be that their better overall midwifery experience, which extends back for twenty years, arises from being genetically and socially more homogeneous than the British, and that they may be constitutionally less liable to the risks of perinatal difficulty.

As things are at present, if I had to advise anyone close to me, I should suggest that she had her pregnancy supervised pre-natally by a family doctor experienced in midwifery, with attendance two or three times at a maternity unit where she is to be confined, and request that, provided her pregnancy and delivery were uncomplicated, she should return home a after 48 hours in the maternity unit, to be cared for by her family doctor and midwife. I think that would meet nearly all the emotional requirements, and avoid nearly all the avoidable risks.

Cot Deaths. I am discussing these here, not because of any public controversy, but because there is at last a faint show of light on the dark distress of the problem; and because, if present results are confirmed, it will need an alteration of the way in which both parents and doctors respond to some of the

Cot Deaths

symptoms and illnesses of young children.

The tragedy hits when a baby or young child, who has not been considered seriously ill, is found dead in its cot. A few cases will be found to have suffocated on too soft a mattress, or an unwisely used pillow. Some others will have had a rapidly fatal pneumonia; but for the majority, no cause will be found, so uncertainty is added to the parents' misery.

A large Department of Health investigation is going on and its report cannot be expected before this edition is printed. I am working from some interim results published in November 1978, from which it seems that roughly thirty unexpected deaths of children under two years occur every year, for every million of the population. What has been found so far is that nearly half these children had symptoms of certain kinds, usually for days rather than hours before death, whose importance had not ben recognised. These symptoms were of a kind which might well prompt contact with a doctor, but which would not be thought of as having any desperate significance — indeed, they also occurred in groups of children similar to the victims, but only a quarter as often. That makes the response to such symptoms difficult to manage, for they are common, and most of them will not have serious consequences. Nevertheless, there seems to be no choice but to bring them to medical notice when they start, knowing that twice as many cot deaths arise in children with such symptoms as in those without them, and that if all children with the symptoms are brought under close supervision, it may prove possible to reduce the number of cot deaths. The symptoms are these:

Cough
Rapid breathing
Wheeze

Cold (not snuffles)
Noisy breathing

Diarrhoea(greater than one loose stool)
More than one vomit
Unusual drowsiness
Irritability and excessive crying

Altered character of cry
Off feeds
Fever
Excessive sweating

Now, it can be seen that assessing every case that shows any of these signs will mean a lot of work for the medical services; and it is really important to behave responsibly. Do let your doctor know as soon as one or more of these symptoms arise. Don't wait until your husband comes home to decide whether to send for the doctor. If you do, you will have a tired doctor for what may be a very delicate exercise of medical judgement; and the patient will lose several hours of treatment. Call the doctor early, and give a clear message.

Whooping Cough Vaccination. In recent years, many family doctors have had to console some parents whose young babies became severely ill during epidemics of whooping cough, and who reproached themselves that, for what they thought were good reasons, they had not had them vaccinated. In fact, these babies could not have been protected by vaccination at the most vulnerable age, the first six months of life, because, even using the revised early vaccination schedules, vaccination would have started only at three months and ended at six months. They caught whooping cough because fewer of the older children around them had been vaccinated in infancy, and so more of them caught it. The reason for that (one does not say 'the blame for that' when the advice was honourably intended) was the information parents received from a number of sources about the possible dangers of whooping cough vaccination.

Whooping cough is most serious when caught by children in the first year of life, when the death rate is fifty times greater than for older children. The death rate for these babies is about eight in every hundred who catch the disease. At all ages, whooping cough can cause pneumonia, with the rare complication of permanent lung damage, and can cause convulsions, with the rare complication of brain damage.

Of all children under two, between five and ten per

thousand a year experience convulsions, whether or not they have been recently vaccinated, from a variety of causes, not all of which are known. Of these children, a proportion will, by coincidence, have been recently vaccinated against whooping cough, and argument is likely to arise as to what part the vaccination played.

There seems to be no doubt that whooping cough vaccination does, rarely, cause convulsions, and that a small number of these result in damage to the brain. Equally, there is no doubt that vaccination reduces the chance of catching whooping cough and reduces its severity if one does catch it. Children in large families are at greater risk of infection, so vaccination is especially important for them, and for those suffering from heart and lung handicap, provided it is safe.

Every parent wants to know: 'will my baby catch whooping cough if not vaccinated? If he is vaccinated, will he have convulsions?' and we cannot answer. All we can say is that, if vaccinated, or if the community in which he lives is highly vaccinated, he is much less likely to catch it; and that the chance of convulsions is very small, provided children at special risk of convulsions are not vaccinated. The present advice is that the following consitute 'special risk', and prohibit vaccination against whooping cough:

History of seizures, convulsions or brain irritation.
History or family history of epilepsy or disease of the nervous system.
Congenital or other defects.
Any feverish illness, until the patient has fully recovered.
Any reaction to a previous dose. (A course of three doses is required.) It follows from this that any general illness, feverishness, convulsions, screaming, redness or swelling at the injection site, should be notified to doctor or health visitor.
Prevalent poliomyelitis locally.

What is the risk to those who are vaccinated? Reports suggest one case of convulsions in twenty-five to fifty thousand children vaccinated. A London survey a few years ago reported no evidence of permanent brain damage after eighty thousand doses, another in the North West Thames region no cases in fifty thousand doses; in Glasgow from 1961 to 1975 there was no known case of severe brain damage directly attributable to whooping cough vaccination, in the one hundred and eighty thousand who received it. These figures and figures from abroad, which I quote later, are contained in the 1977 Report of the Joint Committee on Vaccination. Some people believe that the risks of vaccination exceed those of catching the disease, and point out that its severity started to decline before vaccination began. They attribute this to improvement in general health, nutrition, social conditions, etc. It may well be so, but I think that as an argument against vaccination it will carry more force when we can report no deaths or serious complications from the disease in a year when it is prevalent; and one must note that the death rate for babies under one year old who do catch whooping cough has not altered much in the last twenty years. (This should not be confused with the fact that *the numbers* of babies catching it did fall steadily from 1955 to 1975 — that is, we had reduced the numbers catching it, but are no better at treating it.)

Why is vaccination not started until three months? Whooping cough vaccine is given along with diphtheria and tetanus vaccines as a 'triple vaccine'. Diphtheria and tetanus vaccine give their best protection if used in the second six months of life. This does not apply to whooping cough, and the lower protection against diphtheria and tetanus is considered acceptable, in order to gain the advantage of earlier whooping cough vaccination. At an earlier starting age than three months, diphtheria and tetanus protection would be inadequate.

To summarize: Convulsions, occasionally leading to brain damage, are a hazard of early childhood; most of them caused by disease or injury. Most people believe that the proportion attributable to whooping cough vaccination is small. If, after considering the size of the risk — one in one-hundred thousand doses in West Germany, four cases in Holland between 1962 and 1976, four cases in New Zealand in the same time, and after discussion with someone whose knowledge and judgement you trust, you cannot agree to run that risk, do not let that prevent you from accepting diphtheria, tetanus, polio and measles vaccination. The thought of a return of poliomyelitis or diphtheria is frightening, and the vaccination rates are too low for safety.

Alphabetical Section

Abortion (see also *Miscarriage*), strictly, means the interruption of pregnancy by natural hazard or by surgical or criminal intervention. The former is described under *Miscarriage*.

The operation of terminating pregnancy, if performed during the first three months by an experienced surgeon, is usually simple and requires only a few days in bed. Even so, there are occasional complications and, very rarely, fatalities. Complications are more likely and more severe at the hands of the semi-skilled, and can confidently be expected as the result of amateur attempts. After three months, termination requires an abdominal operation.

Since 1968 it has been legal to produce abortion in a hospital or nursing home registered for the purpose if two doctors agree that it is necessary to protect the life or health (physical or mental) of the mother or of her existing children, or if there are grounds for believing that the baby may be abnormal. (See *German measles*.)

Abrasion. The removal of the outer layers of the skin by contact with a rough surface, as when falling with outstretched hand, or when a falling object deals a glancing blow to the shin. The skin should be gently cleansed with warm *isotonic saline* or by 1 per cent cetrimide (see *Antiseptics*), covered with a single layer of parrafin gauze (see *Dressings*), and a *proflavine cream* dressing applied. The dressing may be changed once or twice daily until healing occurs. If pus forms on the raw area, the doctor should see it. An abrasion which may be contaminated with dirt or soil should be seen by the doctor the same day (**S**), as antitetanus or antibiotic treatment may be called for.

Abscess. A collection of pus in any part of the body; caused by germs or infected matter carried in the blood stream or beyond the capacity of a family doctor. The latter obviously includes referral to the nearest Accident and Emergency Department, or to a simpler casualty department nearby, if one exists, and if it is judged to have the facilities to deal with the case.

In several towns, the old casualty departments of local hospitals have survived, catering for minor casualties; but the situation has been overtaken by a later development. The introduction of levels of pay broadly related to the work done has made it financially impossible to staff some small casualty departments, and they have had to be closed, often to the resentment of those accustomed to use them. Others have been kept open by nursing staff in the nearby hospital volunteering to be available when a casualty arrives, and by general practitioners attending a department by rota, as a voluntary extension of their services to the locality. Elsewhere, junior medical staff employed in other work in the hospitals have agreed to provide services for minor casualties.

Difficulty arises in manning X-ray Departments out of hours; in some towns, X-rays cannot be obtained outside normal working hours, because the radiographers live at a distance. Such a hospital could deal with more serious casualties (broken wrists, ankles and ribs) during the day, but at night would have to forward them to the nearest Accident and Emergency Department.

When a local minor casualty department exists, a considerable number of people present themselves for treatment which their general practitioners are under contract to provide, either during surgery hours or immediately, if they judge the case requires it. Although this group of patients regards attendance at a local casualty department as a matter of ancient right, it is doubtful if there is any compulsion on the N.H.S. to maintain such a facility, when arrangements exist for its provision by the Family Practitioner Service. These arrangements include visitors, and people not on any doctor's list, whom doctors undertake to treat in emergencies. The name of a doctor on call can usually be had from Telephone Enquiries, or the Police Station.

Why Hospital Casualty Departments Close

In the late 1940s, the effects of a number of changes which were to influence Casualty Services began to be felt. Until then, most hospitals maintained permanently staffed Casualty Departments of varying quality, which provided treatment for victims of accident or illness, who did not have a general practitioner, or who could not incur the expense of consulting one.

At that time, most cases attending Casualty Departments were minor, often similar to those attending a doctor's surgery, and were easily dealt with by nursing and junior medical staff within the limited range of diagnosis and treatment then available.

The increasing number of serious injuries, arising from road traffic accidents and mechanization, coincided with advances gained from war experiences, and the snowballing scientific discoveries of the 1930s, to produce a situation in which smaller hospitals could not provide the more developed services and specialist skills needed, if a greater proportion of the seriously injured were to be salvaged and returned to useful life. As a national policy, these skills and high cost equipment were concentrated in centres serving populations of the order of 200,000, a change made possible by free and comprehensive ambulance transport, and involving unavoidable inconvenience and discomfort to casualties who were far from Accident and Emergency Departments.

From the start of the N.H.S. in 1948, everyone became entitled to free general practitioner service, and part of the minor casualty work hitherto done at hospitals became the responsibility of the patient's general practitioner, who now undertakes in his terms of service to treat his patients with the priority which he judges the case to demand, and to advise and if necessary procure, any treatment which he believes to be introduced through a wound. It differs from a *boil*, in which the germs have been rubbed into a hair-root from the surface of the skin, though it may arise from a boil if the latter has been squeezed or mishandled, breaking the barrier which the body's resistance is laying down.

An abscess is painful, and causes feverishness. If near the surface, there will be tenderness, redness, and swelling, and the area will feel warmer than the surrounding skin. Treat by *hot bathing* to the tender area, except for dental abscess. This is a painful throbbing swelling of the face and gum round a tooth and the gum should be treated with hot *normal saline* mouthwashes every hour until the dentist can be visited (same day) and the skin left alone.

Poking and squeezing must be avoided. Pain may be eased with *aspirin* or *paracetamol*, but medical aid is usually needed the same day.

Acne. A combination of enlarged pores, blackheads, red spots, small boils, etc, usually on the face, sometimes on the shoulders and chest. Most common during adolescence and probably caused by increased activity of grease glands in the pores of the skin, producing plugs of waxy matter. These can become infected by germs and fungus from the scales of *dandruff*. Certain foods are thought to make acne worse, in particular cocoa butter (in chocolate) and pork fat. Sunlight helps to heal it.

Treatment **1** Regular de-greasing of the skin, using hot water, a facecloth, and a mild soap, such as Castile. (Some cases will need sulphur soap or lotions but this should be on medical advice.) Ten minutes should be set aside for this each night. The facecloth is loaded with really hot water, lightly smeared with soap, then applied with the flat of the hand as if poulticing the face, renewing soap and water frequently and *never rubbing*. Particular attention should be given to the hair margin, the nasal folds, and behind the ear lobes.

After this, any prominent blackheads are gently pressed on with a comedo expressor (bought from the chemist), a minute spoon with a hole through which the waxy matter escapes. They should *never be squeezed*. The face is then rinsed gently

with plenty of cold water and dried by dabbing with a soft towel.
2 Prevention of secondary infection of the skin by dandruff. This is explained under *Dandruff*.
3 To prevent re-infection, two sets of pillowslips, towels, and facecloths should be used, to allow each set to be boiled after 24 hours use, or longer intervals as the condition improves.

Many cases will respond well to this routine but failure after two or three weeks means that the doctor should be consulted (C).

Addiction to Drugs. Increasingly called *drug* dependence, which describes it more clearly. An addict is a drug taker whose body can no longer do without the drug, and who develops physical illness of varying severity if deprived of it. Also, he usually finds that the dose of drug needed increases steadily. Drugs vary in their power to produce dependence, as do people in their tendency to develop it. Heroin (diamorphine) produces dependence quickly in almost everyone who takes it, with rapid physical and moral collapse; whereas cannabis ('pot') is claimed not to cause dependence, and there is argument as to its adverse physical effects. This has led to a campaign for the relaxation of control on cannabis, but in the present state of public and official opinion that is unlikely to happen, and we should address ourselves to the situation as it is.

Many young people are introduced to cannabis and 'pep' drugs (varieties of amphetamine); a proportion try them and of these a small number become regular users. It is likely that people of defective personality or who are under emotional stress will form the bulk of these, and this vulnerable group of adolescents thus enters a circle where users and pushers of 'hard' drugs will be encountered.

The suggestion that contact with hard drugs would be avoided if use of cannabis were allowed could hardly be extended to amphetamines, which are undoubtedly socially and physically harmful. It is surely preferable to bring those who need help — and who are trying to meet their need with drugs — into touch with a sympathetic doctor or social counsellor.

Addiction to Drugs 39

Adolescence can be a trying time for the teenager and his or her family, and it may be difficult to decide whether irregularity of behaviour is indicative of drug-taking. One should look out for:

1 Regular alterations of mood at or in the course of the weekend, perhaps with peaks of excitement on Friday or Saturday nights, followed by morning apathy.
2 Sleeping out, and unexpected absences from home.
3 Anonymous telephone calls, from contacts seeking or offering supplies.
4 Blood spots on shirt sleeves, or needle marks on the backs of the hands.
5 Spent matches in bathroom or lavatory, which have been used in preparing injections.
6 Noticeable loss of appetite.
7 A peculiar twitching of the lip, reminiscent of a rabbit, has been described in amphetamine addiction.

A parent who finds that her son or daughter is concerned with drugs will be exceptional if she can immediately react with the necessary compassion. More often, shock and anxiety will provoke anger. The situations discovered vary from simple intellectual curiosity to gross mental illness; and anger will worsen all of them, perhaps irreparably. Try to enfold the problem in family sympathy, so that the victim can be strengthened by understanding and support. This is very important, for it must be admitted that shortage of personnel and finance at present make the official arrangements for treatment variable, and a great deal of support will be needed from the patient's family and family doctor, who should be consulted as soon as possible (S).

It is being suggested that some addicts suffer from a gene defect which prevents them from responding to stress by forming ascorbic acid (vitamin C) in their livers, and makes them less able to combat stress. Arising from this, it is now rumoured that 'the thing' for any addiction is to take a lot of Vitamin C; but there is more to it than that, and the treatment will require medical supervision if it is found to be of use.

40 Adenoids and Tonsils

The first step for any sufferer is to get in touch with a sympathetic doctor or social counsellor.

Adenoids and **Tonsils**. Often thought of as a disease, these are useful parts of the body. They form the main parts of a ring of protective tissue at the back of the mouth and nose; adenoids above, a tonsil on each side. Germs in the inspired air are often prevented from reaching the lungs or bronchial tubes by being caught in this ring. Once there, the battle is fought out in the tonsils until the body's powers of resistance overcome the infection. At about the time a child starts school, these organs are approaching their greatest activity and size. This is fortunate, as he needs all the help he can get in combating the various infections to which he will be exposed while his system develops immunity. The adenoids may enlarge to such an extent that they obstruct the airway through the back of the nostrils, causing mouth breathing and poor speech; or allow infection to spread outwards towards

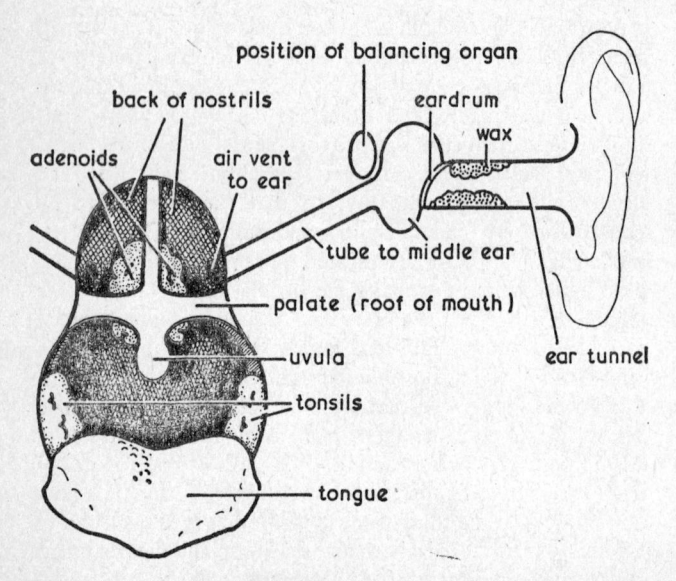

Parts of the mouth and ear.

the eardrums, leading to repeated ear infection (see *Earache*). They then need surgical removal.

The tonsils may collect more germs than they can overcome, so that they are permanently infected and give rise to repeated sore throats. Some of the infection overflows into the *'glands'* of the neck which become swollen and painful. Left to themselves and given one or two fine summers, they may still overcome the infection, but before that happens, the repeated attacks may interfere so much with the patient's education that removal of the tonsils is advised. (See *Tonsilitis*.)

Alcoholism. (see also *Intoxication*). Anyone whose system has become so accustomed to alcohol that it cannot work without it is a chronic alcoholic — in fact, a drug addict. He differs from a heavy drinker in that the latter can stop drinking without becoming physically ill, though he may find the deprivation very unpleasant. A heavy drinker is usually much more open than an alcoholic; broadly, he drinks because he likes it, while the alcoholic drinks because he has to — to help him meet the strains of life at first, and finally because he can't function without it. The finding of a store of empty bottles is often the first hint of chronic alcoholism, and then by careful observation one may recognize the early signs of bleary eyes, shaky hand, and shaky careful 'old man's' signature, before any of the later ones are apparent. Some of the earlier signs, such as leaving one's post temporarily, day or half-day absenteeism, mood changes after lunch, and lowered quality of work, are more noticeable at the place of work, and it is questionable whether the sense of loyalty which may lead colleagues to 'cover up' for the patient is in his best interest.

Every effort of affection and relationship should be exerted by those close to the patient to get him to his doctor with the true history of events. Many alcoholics are adept at concealing and denying their drinking, and this is one of the situations in which the doctor should be apprised of the extent of the discovery before seeing the patient. The doctor will need all the help he can muster in persuading the patient to put himself under expert care, in order to start on the long road home.

Successful treatment of alcoholism usually requires that the patient should never take alcohol again after he is cured. Those close to him should never offer him alcohol. If he is entertained socially, he should be offered a choice of soft drinks in the same tones as others are asked their choice. In this connexion, it would be no bad thing if it became accepted as a mark of bad manners to press anybody once he had declined the offer of a drink.

Literature on alcoholism and its treatment is available from the National Council on Alcoholism, 3 Grosvenor Crescent, London SW1X 7EE. Send stamped addressed envelope for list and prices.

Alcoholics Anonymous. Groups of people who have recovered from alcoholism and make themselves available to help other sufferers. The nearest group can be reached through the local telephone directory. *Al Anon* is a related group for relatives of alcoholics.

Allergy. Many suffer from one form or another, and the tendency often runs in families. As usually understood, it implies a harmful reaction by a part of the body to some substance (food, dust, or contact) to which it has become sensitive. Common forms are *asthma, hay fever, nettle rash* (urticaria), and *eczema* or *dermatitis*. Often the contact responsible cannot be traced; if it is, and can be avoided, no further treatment is necessary. Otherwise, medical advice will be needed.

Alopecia. Loss of hair from any part of the body; most obvious and disturbing when the scalp is affected. In the commonest form, alopecia areata, circular bold patches appear without any inflammation of the scalp. In almost every case, new hair grows after the patch has reached a certain size — which cannot be forecast. When growth restarts, it does so without the need for treatment. Alopecia areata is not infectious, but may be confused with ringworm of the scalp — much rarer — which is. The doctor's advice should be sought to be sure of the diagnosis (C). In severe cases, steroid injections may be advised.

A more serious alopecia, with the loss of all the body hair, sometimes permanently, is a very rare condition.

The cause of the 'natural' thinning or balding which affects middle-aged men and sometimes women at the menopause is not fully understood; there may be a hereditary factor. The treatment of baldness by hair grafts is being developed; advice should be sought from a Member or Associate of the Institute of Trichologists, (MIT or AIT), who work to professional standards (228 Stockwell Road, London, SW9).

(See also *Baldness*.)

Anaemia. Not so much a complaint as a diagnosis, reached by the doctor after hearing the patient's story and examining him. Tiredness and loss of strength may be caused by it, but also by many other things — often by nervous fatigue. In anaemia the blood's power to carry oxygen round the body is reduced by lack of red blood corpuscles. The common causes are inadequate intake or absorption of iron, and repeated loss of small quantities of blood, as from *haemorrhoids*, excessive *menstruation*, a gastric or *duodenal ulcer* or continued self-medication with aspirin. Anaemia is not a suitable subject for home diagnosis or treatment.

The main sources of iron in the diet are red meat and green vegetables. Spinach is not particularly rich in iron, and those who like it should continue to eat it for that reason only.

Angina. This usually refers to angina pectoris, now called angina of effort. It is a pain coming on with exertion, usually felt in the centre of the chest and spreading to shoulder and arm — more often the left. When the patient rests the pain eases. Several conditions can produce similar pain, but true angina is caused by narrowing of the arteries supplying the heart muscle, so that the heart can't meet fully the demands made on it during exertion. The patient should see his doctor so that the course can be found, treatment arranged and advice given. Some re-arrangement of activity may be advised, with regular exercise suited to the patient's condition, and the patient may be urged both to stop smoking and cultivate tranquillity — doubly difficult!

Most victims are relieved by the use of tablets or capsules

taken when pain starts, and increasingly successful surgery is now being practised for suitable cases. Any sudden worsening of angina is a warning to sit quietly at home, avoiding stair climbing, and to ask the doctor to call (D or U). This applies also to any sudden shortness of breath on exertion. (See *Diet*.)

Animals, domestic. Diseases caught from these are numerous; some rare and obscure, some common, such as fungus infection of the skin (see *Ringworm*). Many people are allergic to animals or animal products, and papular urticaria is an interesting skin rash mimicking chickenpox, caused by allergy to the bites of fleas or ticks from animals or birds.

Parrots and budgerigars can spread psittacosis (parrot disease), and illness in either of these birds calls for a veterinary opinion, especially if parrot disease is prevalent. Pigeon fanciers are aware that a small percentage of them run the risk of 'pigeon fancier's lung' caused by allergy to pigeon products; and the same proportion of those keeping budgerigars develop similar trouble. Persisting cough, wheezing or increasing breathlessness on exertion, should alert pigeon or budgerigar owners to the need for a full investigation — sooner rather than later, as after a time the lung damage becomes permanent. (C).

The main object of this note is to call attention to the importance of having cats, kittens, dogs and puppies properly treated by a veterinary surgeon for the removal of worms and other parasites before taking them into the home. Such infestation is common, and can cause serious disease and disability to anyone handling the animal, or by contact with fouled ground — particularly urban parkland. Hand washing with soap and hot water should be the rule after contact with any pet or its quarters, and is particulalry important before meals in a home where pets are kept.

Ankle, twisted (see *Sprain*).

Antiseptic. A substance which kills harmful *germs*. If the germs are inhabiting a patient, any antiseptic used must be harmless to human tissues, and this narrows the field severely.

The use of antiseptics in home treatment is now very limited. *Abrasions* may be treated with diluted cetrimide (see below) followed by *proflavine cream* or with hypochlorite liquids such as 'Milton' following the instruction on the bottle, and the latter are a good treatment for single small boils, which can sometimes be aborted if dabbed two or three times a day with neat 'Milton'. Hydrogen peroxide, '20 volume' strength, one part diluted with three parts of warm water, is a good mouthwash for inflamed or septic gums, and may be used two or three times a day while waiting to see the dentist.

It may be recalled here that soap itself is one of the best antiseptics when used with hot water to maintain a healthy skin in a germ-free condition. It should not be used in the presence of eczema or dermatitis.

A solution of cetrimide 1 per cent in warm water makes a good routine scalp wash for the control of dandruff, and for the management of some other superficial septic conditions of the skin — for the latter it is best used on medical advice.

It is seldom that anyone runs a nail or other sharp object into himself without being subjected to an application of antiseptic to the skin surrounding the puncture. It should be clear that any germ introduced has been deposited deeply in the wound, whose sides close as the nail is withdrawn so that nothing applied from the outside will penetrate. Puncture wounds should be dressed with clean gauze, lint, or linen and seen by a doctor who may decide that antibiotic or other treatment is needed (S). Even the smallest puncture wound of abdomen, chest, head, or near a joint should be seen by a doctor the same day, as the size of the skin wound is no guide to its depth.

'Milton' is now widely used in the sterilization of babies' feeding bottles. Its effectiveness depends on following closely the instructions given in the maternity department or by the midwife. If in any doubt, ask your chemist for the maker's instructions.

Antrum (see *Sinus*).

Anxiety, excessive. Fear is aroused by the unfamiliar, and by anticipation of unpleasantness. It is the natural mechanism for alerting the body in the presence of possible danger, and concentrates the brain on the situation which has produced it. At the same time, a change is produced in the balance of the two nervous networks of the body, closing down unneeded activity — digestion, for instance — and alerting heart, lungs, and muscles so that the brain can select whichever of the well-known trio of fright, flight, or fight seems to offer the best chance of survival. Of these, only fright does not involve the dispersal of keyed-up forces in physical action, and it looks like the worst choice of the three. Nevertheless, this is the state in which a person taking executive decisions usually finds himself in contemporary life, and some of the executive's troubles of heart and circulation may be attributable to the effect of unfulfilled calls for physical activity.

It will be understood that in its original and most useful role fear was a short-lived sensation, ending when the difficulty which provoked it was over. Continuing fear associated with unsolved problems and their consequences is an experience outside the range of its original use, and may produce anxiety *neurosis* in a person constitutionally disposed to it, or in one who is under other forms of stress, particularly frustration, or a conflict between desire and duty in his or her sexual or family affairs. The part played by continuing fear in producing anxiety neurosis is important, as it is the only one which the victim can alter. He cannot alter his inherited constitution, and if his family or sexual difficulties were easily soluble they would not be giving rise to stress.

The first step is to decrease the load of unfinished business the mind is carrying. If the desk worker is one of the chief victims, he also has one advantage — he has a desk. He must now recognize that writing was invented to ease the lot of civilized man, and provide himself with clip boards, paper, and coloured pens. At the start of each day the day and date are written large across the top of one sheet and those of the two following days on two others. The sheets are ruled into two columns, narrower left, wider right. All matters outstanding from the previous day are entered by short titles in the left hand column, and the action needed that day opposite them on the right. The post and matters arising from it are then attended to. Anything for action the next or following day is entered on the appropriate board, though some people prefer to use only one board — TODAY — and to mark 'Carry forward until blank day' as the appropriate action. As the day proceeds the titles of completed items are struck through in red and at the end of the day all titles outstanding are transferred to tomorrow's board. This scheme can be adapted to most jobs which entail decision making, though when the employment is, for example, on a site, the documentation will have to be more portable and less formal. The use of a portable tape-recorder should be considered by anyone who does business while travelling, as letters and instructions can be dictated at the time they are decided on, and are then out of mind for the day. An added advantage of setting out the day's work each morning is that when one comes to a particular item later, one often finds that one's brain has been considering it unconsciously since it was first written, and will produce the answer without further effort — a ploy which is well known by examination candidates.

Someone with a particular constitutional tendency may develop anxiety neurosis under stresses arising only in the family or sexual aspect of life. This is more likely to happen to a family woman, for whom work, family, and sex life are far more intermingled, and whose working life in particular can seem to fill the whole waking day. She will gain help fom the practice of *contemplation*, and from a modification of the memo scheme described above. Advice may be needed from a *marriage guidance* counsellor, or from a doctor if the marriage is not being sexually fulfilled. (See also *Depression* and *Neurosis*.)

Aperient. The best natural aperient is water. A glass should be drunk (hot or cold to taste) on waking and on two further occasions during the day, mid-morning and afternoon. A breakfast food containing bran should be taken, mixed with other cereal if desired; a proportion of the bread eaten should be wholemeal, and use may be made of the laxative properties of prunes and dried apricots. If these fail, and provided that sufficient time has been spent at a regular hour each day for the bowel to act, one should seek medical advice before resorting to regular use of other aperients. If a habit of constipation has developed, it may be necessary to spend up to ten minutes in the lavatory in a relaxed frame of mind, perhaps reading a book, daily for several days before a good bowel habit is established. For occasional use, when temporary constipation follows a disturbance of routine, one, two, or three Senokot tablets may be taken at night to act the next morning. If senna pods are preferred, from six to eight are soaked for three or four hours in half a tumbler of *cold* water, the water (not the pods) being then drunk at bedtime. For use in the morning, effervescent health salts have a mild laxative effect, taken as directed on the container, or half to one level teaspoonful of Epsom Salts taken with a little warm water acts more strongly. (Sufferers from *migraine* sometimes find this useful if an attack threatens.)

No aperient should ever be given in the presence of abdominal pain. It can cause an inflamed appendix to burst.

Any sudden alteration in the bowel's habit of action calls for medical advice.

(See also under *Constipation*.)

Appendicitis, acute. Inflammation of the appendix, a finger-shaped organ in the right lower abdomen. (See illustration, p. 155.)

In a typical attack, pain begins around the navel and after a variable number of hours moves to the bottom right-hand corner of the belly, getting more severe. There may be nausea, sometimes vomiting, and occasionally diarrhoea. Sometimes the pain reaches a climax and then stops, only to return after an hour or two. This usually means that the appendix has perforated, so that peritonitis is brewing, and is by no means the good sign it is sometimes taken for (U).

There is a great variation in the symptoms and signs of acute appendicitis, particularly in children, and the procedure outlined in *Pain, abdominal*, should be followed without hesitation. *Never give an aperient to anyone with abdominal pain.*

Arthritis (Rheumatism of a Joint). There are two common forms, rheumatoid and osteo-arthritis. Rheumatoid often

Arthritis (Rheumatism of a Joint)

affects the wrists and small joints of the hands and feet. Its diagnosis and treatment are matters for the doctor, but one may note its marked tendency to vary in severity, not only from patient to patient (so that one may suffer only inconvenience and another a severe disability), but also from time to time in the same patient; together with the suspicion that a setback is sometimes related to nervous tension, particularly prolonged frustration. The hope that cortisone treatment would provide a cure has unhappily faded, though it still plays a part in treatment, and high dosage of aspirin under medical supervision is now much used.

Osteo-arthritis (the newer name is osteoarthrosis) often affects single larger joints, but also sometimes scattered knuckle joints, in those of over middle age, with loss of the smooth working surfaces of the joint. The cause is disputed, though it can arise from former injury, and, once present, can be made worse by repeated minor injury or misuse of the joint. In the knee joints, this includes long kneeling, particularly out of doors, and having to meet the impact of an overweight body with each walking step. Shedding excess weight helps; also strengthening of thigh muscles to increase their contribution to the act of walking, so sparing the joints from some of the effects of impact. This is done by the regular practice of quadriceps exercises:

1 Sit on edge of table with legs hanging down, thighs supported on table, feet clear of floor.
2 *Slowly* raise the right foot until the leg is straight, taking about five seconds. At the end tighten the knee cap to give a slight 'locking' effect. After two or three seconds, slowly lower the leg to the hanging position, taking five seconds, at the same time raising the left leg to the 'locked straight' position.
3 Repeat the cycle.
4 The exercise should be worked up until six to twelve cycles are being performed two or three times each day. It should not be hurried.

When arthritis of any kind affects the hands, do not turn

taps, etc, by moving the fingers. The fingers should be used to 'lock' the palm on to the tap, like the head of a spanner, and the turn made by moving the forearm, keeping fingers and wrist locked.

The above notes are written to show that self-help can considerably alleviate many cases of rheumatism. The condition should always be subject to diagnosis and advice by the doctor in the first instance (C).

The Arthritis and Rheumatism Council, 8/10 Charing Cross Road, London, WC2, issue booklets *Rheumatoid Arthritis* and *Osteoarthritis*, available free *through your doctor only* (take him two stamped envelopes).

Artificial Insemination. An application to man of the established farming practice whereby semen from a stud bull is distributed over a wide area for the fertilization of breeding cows without the necessity for physical coupling.

The hopes of the more simple-minded of us that this would allow some wives of sterile partners to experience some of the joys of motherhood have been modified by legal and religious objections. The legal position is understood to be that artificial insemination with semen from a man other than the husband (ie, from a donor) is adultery, and a child so conceived a bastard. There can be no objection to its employment, in a more limited way, to convey semen from a husband physically incapable of intercourse to his wife's womb.

Artificial Respiration. It is far better to have had practical training than to try to learn from written instructions. Those who have mastered a method will use it. Those who have not should use mouth-to-mouth respiration, which is the easiest to follow from written description. With all methods, do not waste time; set to immediately.

Mouth-to-mouth method: Lay the patient on his back, face upward. Make sure mouth and throat are not obstructed by dentures, weed, vomit, etc. *Bend head well backwards*, to open the breathing passages. Take a deep breath in, close patient's nostrils with one hand, apply mouth to cover that of patient, and breathe out into it. The chest will be seen to rise; remove mouth and allow chest to collapse. Breathe in, re-apply mouth and inflate again. In the first minute, get in about 20 inflations; thereafter, continue at a rate of 12 to 15 per minute. Twelve a minute can comfortably be maintained for half an hour, and this should be done before breaking off briefly to see whether the patient shows any sign of breathing for himself. If he does not, and if none of the early signs of *death* are present, artificial respiration is continued until patient breathes unaided, or until signs of death are obvious.

If anyone else is present, they should be asked to feel and listen for the heart-beat under the left breast, within a minute of starting artificial respiration. If it is absent, cardiac massage is started, as described under *Drowning*. In the absence of help, artificial respiration must be broken off after the first minute long enough to check the heartbeat, then resumed, stopping again for cardiac massage if necessary every six puffs. Note that for children, inflation should only be gentle, and for infants only 'puffed' from the cheeks. In the case of small children, the operator's mouth can cover the patient's nostrils and mouth together.

Difficulty in inflating may be due to the air passages not being open. Get the head *well* back, and if necessary pull forward the lower jaw by its angles, holding it against the top teeth.

Mouth-to-mouth respiration has the advantage over other methods in that it can (and should) be started while a drowned patient is still in the water, if land cannot be reached in under a minute.

There is no reason why one layer of clean cotton or linen cloth, such as a handkerchief, should not be placed between the operator's and patient's mouth, and it makes the proceeding less distasteful in some circumstances.

Aspirin. A well-tried remedy for headache, rheumatic, and other pains. While the majority of people can take from 1 to 3 tablets 3 or 4 times in 24 hours, a few cannot tolerate it, *particularly past or present sufferers from gastric* or *duodenal ulcer*, who should never take it, as it may cause severe bleeding from the stomach, and a few people who are allergic to it (see *Allergy*). The standard 'Aspirin Tablet BP' for adults is of 300 mg strength, as is the soluble aspirin tablet, which some prefer. The tablets may be crushed before swallowing, and the soluble tablets can be taken dissolved in a little water. Aspirin should be taken *with food* or with a few mouthfuls of milk, not on an empty stomach. Aspirin is contained in several popular tablets sold for relief of pain, and anyone unable to take it should consult the pharmacist before buying these. Alternative products containing *paracetamol* are now obtainable.

Dosage for Children: It has been shown that *children up to the age of 2 years tolerate aspirin badly, and are easily poisoned by overdosing*. The official 'Soluble Aspirin Tablet, Paediatric BPC' is 75 mg, one-quarter the strength of an adult tablet. Most proprietary children's aspirin or junior aspirin are 75 mg or slightly more.

In general, it is best to avoid aspirin altogether, except on medical advice, for a child under 6 months. Between 6 months and a year, quarter of an adult tablet, or a paediatric tablet BPC, or one junior aspirin tablet of 75 mg may be given not more than twice in 24 hours, and for not more than 2 days. From 1 to 2 years, half an adult tablet, two paediatric tablets BPC, or two junior tablets of 75 mg, may be given twice in 24 hours for 2 days only. These doses should not be exceeded and are for children of normal weight only. A 3-year-old can be given three-quarters of an adult tablet, three paediatric tablets BPC, or three junior tablets up to 3 times in 24 hours, and the 4-year-old a whole adult tablet, four paediatric tablets BPC or four junior (75 mg) tablets up to 3 times in 24 hours. This is usually enough for children up to 10 or 12 years of age.

A liquid aspirin mixture can be made; but its use has been abandoned as it was found to start decomposing within a few hours of preparation. Elixir of *paracetamol* can be used for children if a liquid is essential, but they can often take powdered aspirin tablets if the powder is 'puddled' in a teaspoonful of rose-hip syrup or something similar.

Although long continued aspirin treatment is used in the medical care of some diseases, it should only be used for the home treatment of occasional pain, and should not be taken for more than a few days without medical advice.

It is likely that alcohol increases the chance of aspirin damaging the stomach, and the two should not be taken together.

Asthma. A widespread disorder of variable severity. During the attack the muscles round the bronchial tubes go into spasm, narrowing the tubes and obstructing the passage of air in and out of the lungs. As the chest muscles are stronger at breathing in than out, the lungs will tend to fill with air which is then expelled with difficulty, giving the picture of short gulping in-breaths and long forced wheezy out-breaths. (S to UU, depending on severity of attack.)

Asthma usually occurs in people of allergic (see *Allergy*) tendency and there is often a family history of one of the allergic complaints. In an asthmatic subject the attack may be set off by a food, dust, or plant pollen to which the patient is sensitive, occasionally by skin contact (as a complication of primula rash, for example) and often by anxiety or family stress. Attacks can also complicate bronchitis, causing asthmatic bronchitis, and these attacks often subside quickly when the bronchial infection is treated with antibiotic.

An asthmatic who knows what substance is responsible may be able to avoid contact with it, or to undergo a course of desensitizing injections, though the latter calls for considerable patience, and even fortitude, and is rarely suitable for young children. If no cause for the attacks can be found, the asthmatic will be provided by his doctor with the treatment best suited to his case — and finding this may involve trial of several things.

Whatever is found most suitable, it will work best if used *early in the attack*. In the absence of medical advice, a tablet of ephedrine hydrochloride (30 mg for adults, 15 mg for children) may be swallowed with a hot drink.

A patient in a severe asthma attack, sitting up straight, with all his neck muscles straining to force the used air out of his lungs, unable to speak more than a word between breaths, needs a doctor urgently (UU). Patients may occasionally be told that they suffer from 'cardiac asthma' or 'renal asthma'.

These are nothing to do with the asthma described above (which doctors call 'bronchial asthma') and treatment for bronchial asthma is not applicable to them. A patient known to suffer attacks of cardiac asthma, and who develops one, should be supported sitting upright with pillows or a backrest and the doctor sent for (UU). The patient may ask for the windows to be open and this can be done, even at the risk of temporarily chilling the air, a guarded *hot water bottle* being put to the patient's feet. If medical help does not come soon, the attack may be somewhat relieved by two or three teaspoonsful of brandy or whisky.

Athlete's Foot. An infection of the skin, usually between two or more toes, by a fungus. The fungus thrives in hot or moist conditions and so is often acquired in changing rooms and swimming pool premises.

The typical appearance is of cracks in the whitened outer layer of the skin through which the pink under-skin can be seen. Recognition is not always easy, as some cases of eczema can be mistaken for it, and for that reason if medical advice is readily available, it should be taken. For home treatment, if there is delay in seeing a doctor, painting daily with 0.5 per cent solution of crystal violet in water is safe, as it will not harm a mistaken case of eczema. It is deeply coloured and will come off on bed clothes unless cotton socks are worn as a protection.

Prevention 1 Exclusion of infected persons from public baths, etc. 2 Wearing of sandals or beach slippers, or special overshoes in public bathing areas, changing rooms, etc.

Backache. The spine is a complicated structure, extending from the skull to the tailbone. The causes of pain in or near it are numerous, and not good subjects for home diagnosis or treatment. Moderate pain from a strain which the patient remembers may subside in a few days if treated as described under **Lumbago**. Persistent or more severe pain needs medical advice — D, S or C, depending on severity.

Backache can be caused by disease of other organs than the spine, and its severity can be increased by *anxiety*, tension and *depression*, turning an inconvenience into a disability.

Many of the cases of backache which defeat both orthodox and 'fringe' medicine are caused by using the back in a way for which it was not designed. The Back Pain Association (Grundy House, Somerset Road, Teddington, Middlesex TW11 8TT) offers advice on prevention of strain and the correct use of the back; and for them, Dr. David Delvin has written *'You and Your Back'* (Pan Books).

Backrest, Emergency. A pillow or bolster tied to an inverted chair, as illustrated, varied as necessary to suit the headboard.

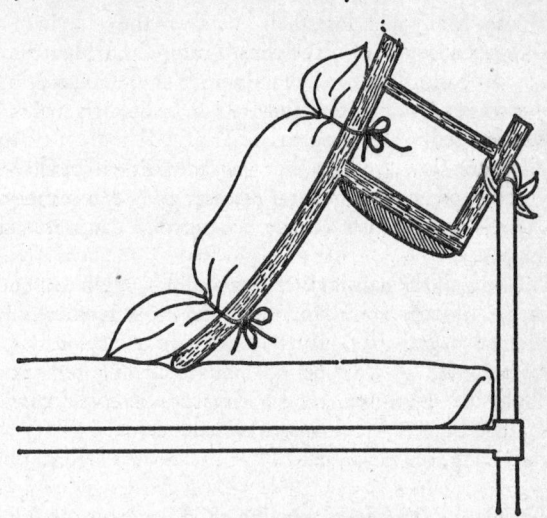

Chair used as a backrest

Backwardness in Children. Very broadly, the following milestones of normal development may be used as a guide:
1 At six or seven months the baby can hold up his head, usually sit unsupported, is beginning to grasp small objects and to respond to close members of the family. Teething usually starts by this time.
2 At one year he is crawling, recognizes faces and voices, makes sounds (not words) and understands some words.

3 At eighteen months he is usually walking, though this may not be achieved until towards the end of the second year.

Should a child not follow this general pattern, the doctor should be consulted (C). It should not cause alarm if he wishes for the further opinion of a children's specialist; the variations within the normal range of development are so large that an expert opinion is often needed. Routine checks on development are now carried out at many Infant Welfare Clinics. (See also *Deafness in children*.)

Baldness. Many men lose their hair from the scalp in middle age, apparently as a result of constitution rather than disease. Some start losing hair earlier, and some keep a full head of hair until old age. A family tendency to lose or keep hair can often be recognized. The progress of 'normal' male balding is usually very slow (years rather than months). Rapid hair loss may accompany some general disease, and requires medical advice. Skin specialists do not believe that dandruff causes balding.

Thinning of the hair is much less common in women but the cosmetic effect is more worrying, and early medical advice should be taken (C). Availability of artificial hair has improved, and it may be possible to arrange for supply through the National Health Service in some cases of premature or severe baldness. For baldness as a disease, and hair grafting, see *Alopecia*.

Bedwetting. The age at which a child becomes 'dry' varies greatly. Most do so during the second and third years. In the great majority of bedwetters, no disease or abnormality is found. All the same, the doctor should be consulted (S), both to make sure that there is no abnormality, and for advice about the management of the problem. (Take a *specimen of urine*.) It is important to avoid scolding or punishment, which aggravate the problem by causing anxiety. The occasional dry bed should be praised, and some small treat arranged, the mother explaining that she can do this in time saved from washing wet bedclothes. The treat should not be too elaborate, for one may find oneself committed to it as the cure progresses! Once a child becomes dry, be prepared for a short setback from illness or anxiety, as when starting school. If handled with patience and reassurance, it usually passes in a few weeks.

Bicarbonate of Soda. This household standby is not as harmless as might be thought; overdosage or continued use can have serious, even dangerous, effects.

Half a level teaspoonful, washed down with a mouthful of equal parts of milk and water during the first half hour of vomiting, may relieve an attack of acute gastritis; and a similar dose will relieve discomfort after an occasional unwise meal. Anyone who has been so unfortunate as to take aboard too much alcohol should summon his resources to take a teaspoonful and wash it down with a glass of water before falling into bed.

At one time favoured as a family remedy at the start of a common cold, it does sometimes seem to relieve symptoms. A level teaspoonful is taken with a flavoured drink three times a day for two days only — not more.

These doses are all for otherwise healthy adults. It is not suitable for children.

Bilious Attack. Usually used to describe vomiting in which yellow or green bile appears in the vomit. This occurs in *migraine*, when the vomiting follows the typical headache, after the first few vomits of an attack of acute *gastritis*, or in intestinal obstruction (see *Vomiting*).

Birth (see *Pregnancy*).

Birth Marks. For a week or two after birth many babies show purplish marks on the brow, face, or back of neck. These are due to pressure on the skin in the process of birth, and clear up without treatment. A 'strawberry mark' is usually present at birth or may appear soon after. It is bright red, raised above the skin, and usually about an inch in diameter. It may increase in size at first, but then slowly shrivels and disappears in the course of a year or two — sometimes longer. It is only seldom that these require active treatment. A 'port wine stain' looks like its description, not raised above the skin, and extending over a larger area. Unfortunately, it is usually permanent, and, as its removal involves plastic surgery and complicated skin grafting, it is usual to mask it with a cosmetic preparation, at any rate until the child is old enough to make a decision about surgical treatment.

Brown or black patches, raised or flat, sometimes with hair on them, are usually called *moles*, under which heading they are discussed.

Blackcurrant Tea. A comforting drink to be taken every four hours or so for a cough. Two large teaspoons of blackcurrant jam (homemade preferably) in a cup, infused with boiling water, stirred for a few minutes, and sipped while very hot.

Lacking jam, blackcurrant puree can be used.

Blackheads (see *Acne*).

Bleeding (Haemorrhage). Leakage of blood from its proper place in the circulation. The body contains about eight pints of blood, most of which is kept in arteries to carry oxygen and nourishment to the various parts of the body, collected by the veins and returned to the heart; sent out on a circuit of the lungs, picking up more oxygen; back to the heart and out through the arteries again. The arterial system is a high pressure supply, the venous system a low pressure return — so low a pressure that the returning blood from the limbs has to be squeezed onwards by the movement of the muscles surrounding the veins (which are fitted with non-return valves to ensure one-way flow).

If the circulation is damaged, escaping blood will flow either out through a wound in the skin (external bleeding) or into an internal organ or tube. The latter is internal bleeding, and may not be suspected unless the blood is expelled from the organ concerned, as when blood is vomited from a bleeding gastric ulcer. Thus much more blood can be lost from the circulation by internal bleeding before the alarm is raised. In external bleeding there is little doubt what is happening, as the blood is seen to be escaping from a cut or wound. If from the high pressure arterial system the blood will come in spurts, keeping time with the patient's pulse. Also, being oxygenated blood it will be bright red. Blood from a damaged vein will be dull in colour and flow steadily without pulsation. Generally blood loss from arterial bleeding is quicker and greater than from a vein, exept that damage to a *varicose vein* in the leg may produce a rapid loss, since the varicose vein has lost its non-return valves and the blood will be expelled under a head of pressure of three or four feet. It stops at once if the patient lies down with the leg raised so that the wound is higher than his head.

The first-aid treatment of bleeding is to stop it, and the simplest way is the best. If a sterile wound dressing is available, it is used; otherwise a freshly laundered (preferably boiled) towel or napkin, or even the inside pages of the day's newspaper may be pressed into service. If possible, fold into a pad so that a surface is exposed which has not touched other objects. The hands should be well washed with soap and water before starting, if time allows. The pad is then pressed on the wound or bleeding point with sufficient pressure to stop the bleeding — clearly it should be sufficiently small to allow observation of this — and the pressure maintained for five to seven minutes. It is then cautiously released and the wound observed. If no more bleeding occurs, replace the pad and bind it in position with a bandage. The patient can then be moved, or move himself, to hospital or a doctor's surgery according to the urgency and site and size of the wound. If bleeding restarts, pressure is reapplied and inspection repeated. If this is not successful in the course of fifteen to twenty minutes, or before if firm pressure has been unavailing, the patient must be put in touch with a trained first aid helper, doctor, or casualty department as soon as possible. Bleeding from hands or arms will stop sooner if the part is raised, and once controlled, a sling should be used (see *Injuries*). *Nosebleed* is dealt with under that heading.

Internal Bleeding. Usually this is reflected in the general condition of the patient, and it is this which brings the need for medical care to notice. A haggard face, the complexion paler than usual, some restlessness, complaint of thirst, and a raised *pulse* rate which increases each time it is taken all indicate the need for help (U or UU). If caused by accident, the bleeding may be into the abdominal cavity or from the site of a major fracture, such as the thigh. As far as possible, without disturbing any injured parts, the patient is wrapped with blankets and supported with words of comfort until skilled help arrives. At this stage it is better to give nothing by mouth.

Bleeding into a hollow organ, such as bladder or stomach, may become apparent when the organ empties. Thus, bloodstained urine may arise from bleeding in the bladder, though this is only one of the causes. It is very seldom serious enough to cause general effects, though the victim may justifiably 'come over queer' when he sees what is happening. Note whether the blood comes out completely mixed with urine, or whether it is present only at the start, followed by clear urine, whether any small clots are passed, whether there is any difficulty in passing urine, and if pain occurs before, during, or after the attack. If possible a few ounces of the first offending urine passed should be saved and taken to the doctor in a clean bottle (see *Specimen of urine*). If the abnormality is noticed too late for this, the next emptying of the bladder should be into a suitable vessel so that a specimen can be saved. Unnecessary alarm is sometimes caused after a heavy intake of beetroot. The doctor or his laboratory will be able to sort this out (S).

More alarming, and with more immediate effect, is bleeding into the stomach, often from an ulcer, sometimes from the effect of aspirin on a susceptible person. The patient vomits half a pint or more (it will certainly seem more) of bloodstained gastric juice — perhaps mixed with his last meal. It may be dark brown or even black, or red if the bleeding has occurred recently, or is continuing. It is obvious that medical help is needed urgently (UU); meanwhile, little can be done except comfort the patient and help him to remain as quite and still as possible, preferably propped up in bed unless the blood loss is so severe that he becomes dizzy, when he should be gradually laid down. The vomit should be saved for the doctor to see.

It will be clear from the above that severe blood loss from the stomach is an emergency. The appearance of flecks or streaks of blood in the vomit in the course of a severe attack of *gastritis* is something quite different, is not usually serious and does not call for emergency measures. On the other hand the *coughing up* of even a small quantity of blood needs full investigation. The patient's general condition is not usually affected, unless an unusually free flow occurs, but the occurrence can be an early warning of severe disease in the chest and the doctor should be consulted (S or D according to severity). Home treatment is only called for in the occasional case who is producing a mouthful of blood with each cough. He should be propped up in bed and be given chips of ice to suck until the doctor can see him (U or UU).

Bleeding from the rectum is usually noticed when passing a motion and can vary from a streak on the toilet paper to a massive loss from a burst haemorrhoid. The latter is rare, but requires bed rest until the doctor can see the patient (U or D, exceptionally UU if massive loss continues) but all cases of rectal bleeding need medical assessment (C).

Bleeding from the womb. A woman who is simply having a heavy period and using, say, twice the usual amount of protection, will not normally be much worried, though it is a situation which she should discuss with her doctor in due course (C). The sudden and unexpected loss of a quantity of blood, often when at toilet, is another matter. The patient should lie down with the foot of the bed or couch raised some six inches, and be warmly wrapped with a guarded *hot water bottle* to the feet. After an hour or two she will probably be able to move about without undue loss, and can consult her doctor later (D, S, or V). If bleeding in quantity notably more than the usual menstrual loss continues, a doctor should be called (U) but if the patient's general condition is obviously worsening, with signs of *shock*, the doctor must be sent for urgently (UU) and if he is not available ambulance or any available transport be used to take the patient to hospital without delay. (See also *Wounds, Dressings.*)

● **If a patient is not within the scope of home care, or**

worsens in spite of it, or if there is any uncertainty, a doctor should be consulted.

Blisters. These can be caused by disease or injury. The former need medical advice; they are usually scattered about the body and not only on those parts exposed to pressure (see *Chickenpox, rash*). If the patient is not feverish or constitutionally ill, it is usually safe to attend the surgery. Otherwise the doctor should be asked to call (**V** or **D** according to severity).

Some people develop blisters, usually on the legs, dome-shaped and about ¼ to ½ in, in diameter, after being bitten by mosquitos or other grass dwelling insects. Preserve the blisters as long as possible, cleansing the skin gently with warm soapy water each day. If they become infected, with throbbing pain and redness spreading to the surrounding skin, attend the doctor (**S**).

Blisters on palms, fingers, soles and toes, are caused by overuse, before the skin has had time to harden, as when starting too enthusiastically to walk, garden or row. To avoid these, allow several days of gradually increasing activity, keep the skin clean with warm soapy water, avoiding detergents, and use any protective gloves and footwear available. Some people rub on surgical spirit each day.

Shoes for walking should be chosen when wearing the correct socks — woollen, and either one pair of thick or two thinner. Once a blister occurs, try to keep it unburst; clean with warm soapy water and protect with a dry *dressing* of gauze. Avoid using that skin area until the skin beneath the blister has had time to harden. If you have to walk or work on or with it, protect it while in use with a layer of stretched Elastoplast then wash the skin gently afterwards and apply a gauze dressing.

Blood Pressure. See under bleeding for a brief description of the circulation of the blood. A person may describe himself as suffering from blood pressure, meaning that the pressure under which the blood circulates is higher than normal. Such an increase is often found in the course of a medical examination and in many cases is of no importance. A serious rise in the circulation pressure can eventually affect the heart or kidneys if not brought under control, and there is risk of leakage from an artery if the pressure exceeds what the artery can withstand. If this happens in the brain, it can produce a *'stroke'*. The majority of cases of raised blood pressure either do not need treatment, or can be brought to a safe level by treatment.

Boil. A boil develops when a *germ*, usually a staphylococcus, is rubbed into a hair root in the skin; so boils are more common where friction of the skin occurs and when there is a source of infection. The latter may occur from a chance contact with someone else infected, or by carriage on the fingers from a reservoir of infection in the patient, most commonly the nostrils, sometimes the buttock cleft or genital area. Fingers which have touched these areas can carry the germs, and if the skin is then rubbed the conditions necessary for boil formation are present. Nostril infection is a cause of recurrent *styes* and it may be necessary to use a course of antibiotic ointment to the nostrils from time to time (C). Anyone whose work involves rubbing any part of the skin should ensure that the part is cleaned daily with soap and water (sometimes the doctor will advise an antiseptic soap — not all skins will tolerate them) and that the underclothing in contact with that part is changed daily, preferably being boiled at each change.

As the germs multiply in the hair root, a spherical swelling is formed which communicates with the skin surface at the exit point of the hair. *Pus* will eventually discharge at this point. The body's defences build a barrier round the developing boil to prevent infection spreading into the tissues, and germ-eating cells are sent in to mop up the infection. Pus consists of these cells, together with germs, in great numbers, and can itself give rise to infection if not disposed of by burning.

Anyone employed in food handling should not work while they have a boil.

Treatment: Hot bathing every two to four hours will bring the boil to a head and allow it to discharge. The bathing is continued until no more pus comes away, then a paraffin

64 Breast

gauze *dressing* is applied daily until healing is complete. Large boils and those on the face need a doctor's advice and possibly antibiotic treatment (S). **NEVER** *squeeze, prick, or press a boil*. It will break down the barrier that has been formed and broadcast the infection, possibly even leading to blood poisoning.

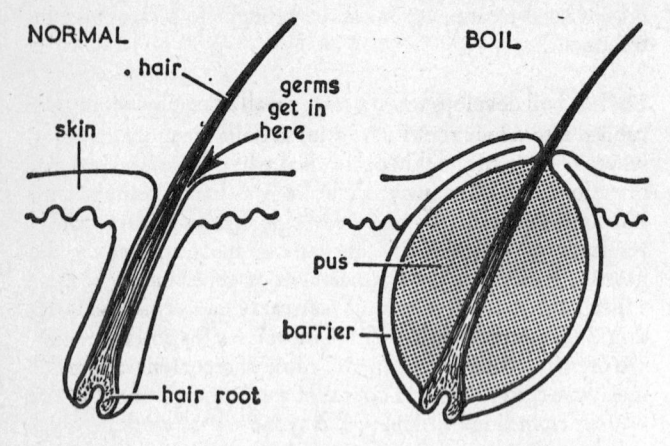

Breast. A lump or swelling in the breast should be seen by a doctor as soon as reasonably possible (S or C). Most of these are not serious, but a few of them are early cancers, and in these the chances of cure are high if treatment is started early. It may be impossible to tell the cause of a lump on simple examination, and the patient should be prepared for her doctor to recommend a surgeon's opinion. If the surgeon has any doubt, he will advise that the lump be removed for examination. It is sometimes possible for this to be done while the patient remains under anaesthetic so that any further operation indicated by the nature of the lump can be proceeded with. (See *screening* about routine examination of your own breasts.)

A general painful swelling of one or both breasts sometimes occurs in the course of *mumps*. The patient should stay in bed taking *aspirin* or *paracetamol* and ask her doctor to call (V).

A hot painful patch, sometimes red and hard, on the breast

of a nursing mother may be caused by inflammation in a blocked milk duct. A *kaolin poultice* is applied to the inflamed area, the breast comfortably supported *from below* by a suitable brassiere and the doctor asked to see it (D, V, or S according to severity). Unless he advises otherwise, feeding from the inflamed breast may continue.

Enlargement of the nipple area on one or both sides is a common temporary feature of normal adolescence in boys. In almost every case it clears up in the course of a few months. Although treatment is both ineffective and inadvisable, it is best to let the doctor see him, to exclude the very occasional case in which sexual development may be amiss (C).

Breath-holding attacks (see under *Convulsion*).

Breathlessness. Those who find themselves short of breath during exertion, either from disease or the effect of age, should use pursed lip breathing, taking in two or three deep breaths quickly, then expelling the air slowly through pursed lips, immediately replenishing and repeating. (This is not a substitute for correct diagnosis and treatment!)

Bronchitis, acute (see *Cough*).

Bronchitis, chronic. An insidious complaint so common in this country that on the Continent it is referred to as the English disease. Though the causes are not accurately known, one factor may be the breathing over a long period of polluted air, particularly air containing sulphur fumes or tobacco smoke. Individual constitution may play a part, and established cases are made worse by exposure to smog, cigarette smoking, and recurrent respiratory infections. The onset is gradual; at first a cough every winter, lasting longer each year, then repeated once or twice in the season; coughing up of *phlegm*, which may be yellow or green, in the morning; increasing shortness of breath when working or climbing. The diagnosis will be made by the doctor, sometimes with the help of X-rays, and the sooner it is made the sooner the progress of the disease can be slowed or halted.

An important measure, and a difficult one to achieve, is to move out of the area of polluted air. Cigarette smoking should be stopped, and a patient given to corpulence should reduce weight — a difficult task if he has also stopped smoking (see *Obesity*). All coughs and any but the mildest colds should be treated promptly (see *Common cold*) and the patient should be immunized before each winter with influenza vaccine.

The treatment of acute attacks of bronchitis by antibiotics may be advised by a doctor, as may the taking of antibiotics in courses or throughout the winter, though the latter is now less in favour. A victim of chronic bronchitis should not go out during a fog and should try to keep it out of his house.

Indoors, the aim should be to keep an even temperature throughout the living area, including passages and lavatory, as far as possible day and night. Some ventilation is needed, but it is easily overdone, and if one can feel a draught it certainly has been. Moistening the air may help, particularly if heating is by radiant sources. A small bowl of water in front of the fire is not enough — two washing up bowls would be better; not necessarily in front of the source of heat, but exposed to the air in different parts of the room.

Bruise. The release of blood into the tissues following injury. This can occur at all levels, but the word is usually used when the released blood is sufficiently close to the skin for its colour to be apparent. The prompt application of a *cold compress* (replacing the beefsteak of earlier days) relieves discomfort and may limit the amount of bruising.

If a limb is involved, it will be less painful if propped level than if allowed to hang down. In the course of a few days, the blood pigment released will change colour to yellow and will be scavenged by the repair cells of the body. The fluid part of the released blood tends to seep downwards, so may produce swelling of the ankle or toes if the leg is bruised, or puffiness of the eyelids from a bruised scalp.

Bunion. A complication of *hallux valgus*, in which the exposed tissues round the great toe joint become thickened. From time to time the swelling becomes acutely inflamed and needs medical care. While awaiting this, *hot bathing* repeated two to four hourly will bring relief.

The pressure of the shoe on a bunion can be relieved by the use of a wooden shoe tree to which a 'dome of silence' has been fixed in the position which the bunion occupies on the foot. (To find this, mark the bunion on the outside of an old shoe with a chalk ring. Drive a tack through the leather into the tree to mark the centre of this ring in the wood. Remove tack, extract tree, and centre the dome of silence on the tack mark.)

Burns and **Scalds.** Although in general a scald is less severe than a burn, as its temperature is limited to that of boiling water, the severity is increased if water soaks clothing which cannot be quickly removed; and this points to a difference in first aid treatment. For a scald, and a corrosive chemical burn, the soaked clothing must be removed in as few seconds as possible, with the aid of scissors if necessary. The remnants of charred clothing in and around a burned area are doing no harm, having been sterilized by the burn, and attempts to remove them will only contribute to infection of the damaged area. Avoidance of this is the main duty of first aid treatment, and dry *dressings*, sterile if available, should be gently applied to cover the whole area, and fixed in whatever way possible. Avoid fluffy material. Apply any padding available *outside* the dressing to absorb exuded fluid.

Pain in small burns and scalds is reduced by holding under running cold water for ten minutes before gently drying and dressing, and there is a suggestion that if done immediately the chilling reduces the extent of damage. It should also be done for burns by chemicals *as soon as possible*. Thereafter the use of *aspirin* or *paracetamol* will help.

Further treatment varies with the extent and site of the injury. Clearly, a quarter inch burn on the hand or finger while cooking is a minor injury, whereas involvement of several fingers with hot fat needs medical aid (S or U). Small blisters are probably best preserved for a few days if possible to allow thickening of the skin layers below, and to guard against infection. Larger ones need medical advice (S or U).

68 *Butterfly Pillow*

Application of antiseptics, powders, oils or grease is no longer recommended.

The object in dressing burns or scalds is to protect from airborne *germs* but allow sufficient ventilation for evaporation of fluid from the area. Too complete a sealing will trap sweat and serum, causing soggy infected tissues and slow recovery. Several layers of sterile gauze secured by bandage or a lattice of plaster are best. In emergency for large areas, laundered sheets and towels will be used, and pillowslips are useful for limbs.

Shock is to be expected if more than 10 per cent of the whole body surface is involved, and such cases should be got to hospital for resuscitation within one hour — less if a large area is involved, when UU. (10 per cent is roughly one thigh, or one upper limb, or the head-and-neck, or one leg with foot. The whole trunk is 36 per cent. The grasping surfaces of the palm and fingers only 1 per cent, so this common and painful burn does not present a shock hazard, though it does need medical treatment to prevent deformity.) While waiting for transport, and on the journey to hospital, a conscious patient should drink half a cup of water every ten minutes to combat shock.

Butterfly Pillow. A pillow so arranged as to allow the head and neck to remain in their natural position on the shoulders

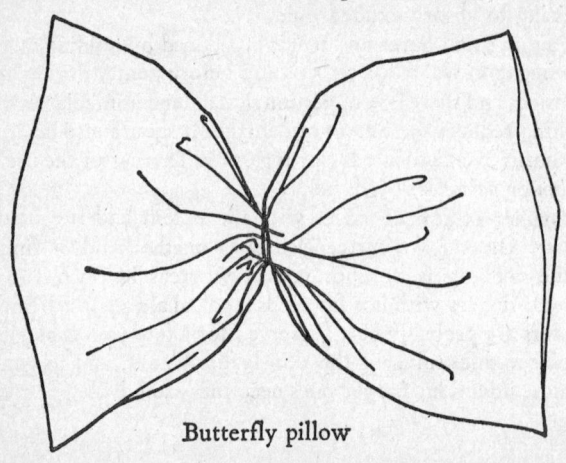

Butterfly pillow

when the patient is lying. A soft pillow is tied around its middle with a few turns of darning wool. It is used by itself with no bolster or under-pillow, the patient's neck lying across the waist of the pillow.

Those who find that the single pillow leaves their heads too low for comfort should raise the head end of the bed four or five inches by means of blocks.

Caesarean Section. Delivery of a baby by an abdominal operation if a normal delivery is impossible, as, for instance, by reason of narrowing of the birth canal.

Cancer. A wide term used to cover all forms of malignant disease — that is, disease (usually a tumour or lump) which spreads into other parts of the body, invading and destroying.

Many cancers are curable if found early enough, particularly those in the following sites: breast, womb, skin, kidneys, bowel; and medical advice should always be sought as soon as possible (S, C) in any of the following circumstances:

Lump in the breast, or any other part.
Vaginal bleeding after the menopause (or before it at other than the usual times).
A spot or sore on the skin, lip, or tongue, which does not heal in a few weeks.
A wart or mole which increases in size.
Coughing blood-stained phlegm; cough or hoarseness lasting more than two or three weeks.
Passing blood in the urine.
Passing blood from the bowel or any change in the usual pattern of the bowel's action.
Difficulty in swallowing, or a feeling that food is held up after swallowing.
Persistent loss of appetite, or indigestion.
Loss of weight.

This does not imply that any of these symptoms mean that the patient has cancer — most will prove not to have, as cancer is only one of the many causes of the symptoms listed — but if everyone sought early advice for these occurrences many early cases would be found and cured.

Prevention of Cancer. Present knowledge has only touched the edges of this subject, and it is probable that the number of *screening tests* will increase in the future. Avoidance of lung cancer by avoiding cigarettes has already been dealt with. Two other points:

1   Recent evidence suggests that cancer of the neck of the womb (cervix uteri) is commoner in women whose husbands are uncircumcised and it is believed that repeated contact with smegma, the greasy secretion inside the foreskin, may be responsible. Scrupulous cleanliness seems to be called for by the husband from the start of marriage. Such wives might reasonably feel the need to make use of cervical smear *screening* at regular intervals.
2   It may be that long-term irritation by food swallowed too hot plays a part in cancer of the gullet. This suggests that the lips should be used more frequently for testing the heat of food and drink and that a mouthful which is found to be too hot is better rejected than swallowed.

Car Sickness (see *Travel Sickness*)

Carbon monoxide poisoning (see *Gas Poisoning*)

Carbuncle. An abscess lying under the skin and eventually bursting through it in several places. It differs from a boil, where the hair-root in which the germs multiply forms a natural barrier and a channel for the discharge of pus. To contain a carbuncle the body's defensive system has to bring up materials to wall it off, and the infection has a chance to spread while this is happening. The result is an angry red dome an inch or more across, very painful and often making the patient feel ill. The use of antibiotics has revolutionized treatment, and the doctor should be given the opportunity to see it as soon as possible (S). On no account squeeze or prick.

Cardiac Massage. A means of restarting the heart when it has stopped after electric shock, drowning, etc. The method available for first aid is external massage and is described under *drowning*.

Carpal Tunnel Syndrome (see *Pain in Hand*).

Carrier. One who, healthy himself, carries germs which can cause disease in others. Convalescents can carry disease for some time after they appear to be cured.

As carriers of *typhoid, dysentery* and *food poisoning* may excrete germs from bowel or bladder, they can contaminate sewage or, in the absence of scrupulous cleanliness of habit, any foodstuffs they may sell or prepare. It has recently been found that many people carry staphylococcal germs, often inside the nostrils, whence they can be carried on the fingers and either contaminate food (see *Food Poisoning*) or cause infection such as boils or even blood poisoning in others. During epidemics of *poliomyelitis* many people are throat or bowel carriers and there are good reasons for avoiding congested meetings at such times.

Once discovered, a carrier needs to cooperate with his doctor or Community Physician in avoiding the spread of infection.

Cataract. Mistiness of the lens at the front of the eye which focuses the vision on to the sensitive retina at the back. It usually occurs in the elderly and is caused by the lens becoming hard and eventually opaque. A patient told that a cataract is present often fears he is destined to be blind, but in the majority, the cataract can be removed by operation, and a powerful spectacle or contact lens then takes the place of the lost natural one, so that objects can again be focused on the retina. The recovery of vision then depends on how well the retina has survived the general process of ageing. A patient often has several years of useful sight from the time when the earliest misting of the lens is noted, and the stage at which an operation is advisable is a matter for the judgement of the eye specialist.

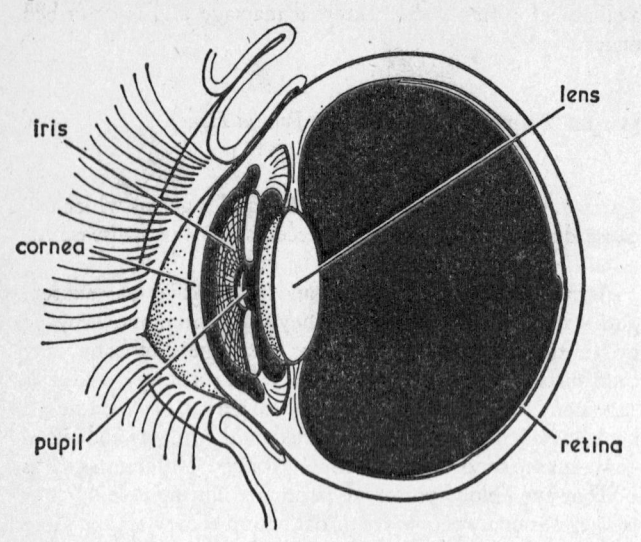

The structure of the eye

Catarrh. A technical medical term which has come to mean something different in ordinary speech. A sufferer may describe as 'catarrh' a condition in which he has a stuffy nose interfering with breathing and is aware of the frequent need to swallow something at the back of his throat.

Stuffy breathing is often due to 'vasomotor rhinitis', a constitutional tendency of the spongy lining of the nostrils to swell. It is worse in relaxing than in bracing *climates*, and is most troublesome when the patient lies down. An attempt to ease this by using a lot of pillows may succeed at the cost of a ricked neck, and it is better to raise the head of the bed on blocks, four to six inches. If the condition happens in summer only, or on exposure to dusts, etc, an *allergy* may be suspected and medical advice sought. A child or young adult very keen to control their rhinitis may try the old remedy of a daily cold bath, having first consulted his doctor to make sure he has no sinus infection or other impediment. The 'catarrh' which is swallowed from time to time from the back of the throat is a natural product, mucus, which is formed in the breathing passages and moved slowly to the back of the throat. Its function is to trap germs and dust in the air intake, and it is swallowed from time to time to be sterilized by the gastric juice in the stomach. Production of, and swallowing of, mucus is a natural process, part of the body's defences, and not a disease. Some people produce more than others and some are more sensitive to the need for swallowing; once they are reassured they usually stop worrying about it.

In the course of a cold or sore throat the 'uvula' (see diagram, page 40), a small finger-shaped object hanging from the arch of the throat, may become swollen and lengthened, particularly overnight, and one then has the sensation of repeatedly swallowing something which reappears. It often improves after a cup of hot tea, or gargling with a teaspoonful of salt in a glass (half a pint) of hot water. If it persists more than a few days, advice should be taken, as it may be kept going by infection in a sinus or antrum (C).

Cerebrospinal Meningitis. A form of *meningitis* particularly prevalent in conditions of overcrowding and massive movement of population — typically in refugee reception areas.

The onset is rapid, with high fever, severe and increasing headache, made worse by light, so that the patient turns away from the window. Bending the head forwards produces pain in the back of the neck or chest. It is obviously a severe illness and medical help is needed (U).

Chickenpox. One of the common infectious diseases usually experienced in childhood. An average attack makes the victim immune to further infection — the occasional second attack usually affects someone who has had a mild attack previously, insufficient to give immunity.

Between two and three weeks after contact with a case, and sometimes after a day or two of headache and backache, scattered red raised spots appear on the trunk, each developing a clear central blister. There may be several 'crops' of spots for the first few days, and the face, scalp and trunk are infected in turn, followed by the limbs, on which spots are less crowded. The blisters change to small scabs in the course of a few days, and if these are allowed to separate naturally they leave little or no trace on the skin. Picking at the scabs will leave scars, and patients need to be warned against this. The spots should be dabbed with calamine lotion every few hours at first, and a dose of aspirin (300 mg for an adult every 4 hours — see under *Aspirin* for children) will also relieve itching. A sore mouth or throat at the start of the illness is due to pocks at those sites. It is usually not severe and disappears in a day or two. Continued isolation of patients until all scabs drop off is no longer advised, and return to school or work is allowed two weeks from the onset.

Chickenpox is not compulsorily notifiable and it will not usually be necessary to call the doctor to each successive case in a family unless illness is severe enough to need advice. Quarantine: about 24 days, but isolation of contacts is not usually practised.

Chilblains. People subject to chilblains develop painful red or purple swellings on fingers, toes, and heels in cold weather — or when there is a sufficiently rapid downward change in the temperature to provoke an attack; thus, after a long hot summer, chilblains may be seen in October, whereas after a cold summer one may not see them until the following January. The cause is not clear, but they seem to be a form of cold injury arising in the circulation just below the skin — in fact, a very mild form of frostbite.

Prevention. Some doctors advise a course of calciferol in the autumn, or the taking of tolazoline tablets throughout the winter. Avoid sudden changes of skin temperature during the winter, by the use of wool socks, double socks if wearing rubber boots, avoiding tight footwear and suddenly heating cold feet on hot pipes, or before the fire. Gloves should be used throughout the winter, even for short outings (to dustbins, etc). Treatment of established or broken chilblains is medical (C).

Chill. As usually used, implies an acute infection, e.g., chill on the bladder, which is *cystitis*. 'Catching a chill' usually means catching a virus infection, such as influenza or one of its lesser brethren. Most of us believe that if we expose ourselves unwisely to cold we develop acute symptoms, usually in the respiratory system; but I understand the expert view to be that we connect the chilling in retrospect with the occurrence of respiratory virus infection, or perhaps that in the early stages of an infection we feel cold more readily.

One form of allergic rhinitis, see *Hay Fever*, is triggered by a chilling of the skin, causing sneezing on moving from a warm to a cold room.

For effects of severe chilling, see *Exposure*.

Choking. Three hundred people die of choking in Great Britain every year. The first aid priority is to send out a call for any available doctor. Meanwhile, look in the patient's mouth. If the food morsel can be seen, try to pick it out with finger or eyebrow forceps. If not visible, do not poke about, as that will wedge it in tighter. Get someone to hold the patient's legs so that he is upside down, then give hard thumps over the shoulder blades until the food is dislodged.

If this fails, the doctor on arrival may have to open the windpipe, so get somebody looking for a razor-blade and pipe stem, or similar short tube.

Even the thumping produces less force than a good cough, provided the patient has kept enough air in his lungs to make one.

Circumcision. The removal of the foreskin which shields the end of the penis, the male sexual organ. Originally a hygienic measure by natives of hot dry lands where water was not available for daily cleansing, it was widely practised in this country until the 1940s, when it fell into disrepute as a mutilating operation unnecessary in conditions of modern hygiene. This latter view assumed that males would have facilities, *and would use them*, for daily cleansing of the penis under the foreskin.

In the absence of this, a natural secretion, smegma,

accumulates and can lead to infection and inflammation of the foreskin which will need medical attention (S). Recent research suggests that there may have been more good in the old practice than was realized, as it seems that repeated contact with smegma can lead over the years to cancer of the womb in the wife of an uncircumcised man who does not practise adequate hygiene. If this research is confirmed, it will follow that:

1 An uncircumcised husband must cleanse the penis daily.
2 Parents of a male child left in his natural state have an obligation to train him in a daily routine of cleansing.
3 Wives of uncircumcised men should avail themselves of regular cervical smear tests (see *Screening*).

A male child is often brought to the doctor in the first year of life, or later, because his foreskin can't be folded back on the penis completely. This is due to late separation of the foreskin and will usually right itself. The opening of the foreskin should be gradually enlarged by pushing it gently back as far as it will go at bath time, then bringing it forwards again. Occasionally, the foreskin when pulled back will get stuck behind the rim of the penis. If it can't be persuaded back

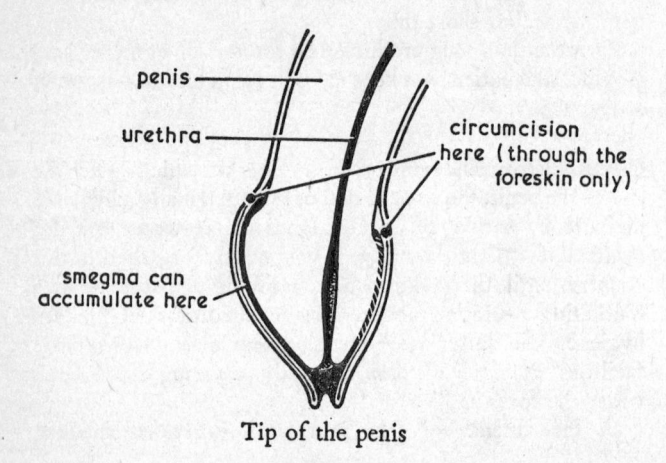

Tip of the penis

(see *Foreskin*), a doctor, nurse, or health visitor should see it *the same day*.

Occasionally, circumcision is needed as a planned surgical operation, to relieve obstruction to the flow of urine or if the foreskin is subject to repeated attacks of inflammation.

Cleft Palate and **Hare Lip.** Parents of a baby born with cleft palate or hare lip can be assured that surgical treatment gives good cosmetic and vocal results in the great majority of cases, although more than one operation may be necessary.

Climate. Many people believe that climate affects their general state of well-being. They recognize 'bracing' and 'relaxing' as the extremes of local climate. In a bracing climate, typically near the East, South East, or eastern part of the South Coast, such people feel alert and vigorous, need less sleep and are able to to work better with body and brain than they are in the relaxing climate of the West Coast or in some inland areas where the free flow of air is baffled by surrounding hills.

On returning from a stay in a more bracing air than they have been used to, many people feel a physical fatigue, unconnected with the end of their holiday, which may last for several weeks.

Cold Feet. The sensation of having cold feet is often due to badly controlled circulation. In older people it may be due to narrowing of the arteries and needs medical diagnosis and treatment. This is also necessary if the condition arises suddenly in younger people; but a life-long tendency is often constitutional, and is attributable to poor control by the nervous system of the circulation in different parts of the body.

Various dodges are used by sufferers, such as the wearing of thick wool socks, and exercising the circulation by taking a short walk before bedtime.

Cold Pack or **Compress.** A cloth wrung out of cold, preferably iced, water and applied to the affected part several layers thick. It is left on, and the process repeated every quarter or half hour.

Cold Sore (see *Herpes Simplex*).

Colic. Surges of painful activity in the muscular wall of any natural tube. It happens when the tube tries to overcome an obstruction, as when a 'stone' lodges in the tube leading from the kidney to the bladder (renal colic); or when the muscles make violent efforts to expel infected contents, as in the commonest form of colic in the lower bowel (see *Gastroenteritis*). Renal colic is felt in one or other loin and the pain extends downwards towards the groin. It is often very severe, the patient pale and sweating and needing a doctor (U). Meanwhile there is not much to be done, though a guarded *hot water bottle* to the loin may bring relief. Gallstone colic is caused by a stone formed in the gall bladder, blocking its exit tube. The severe bouts of pain are felt under the right rib margin and may extend to the right shoulder. Again, a doctor (U) and a guarded hot water bottle are needed.

Coma (see *Unconsciousness*).

Common Cold. 'There are many ways of curing a common cold in a fortnight. If left alone it will go in two weeks.' A fair observation, but some measures can make life more tolerable while the patient's powers of resistance are mustering and overcoming the cold virus. Of these, the writer favours *bicarbonate of soda* for otherwise healthy adults. *A steam inhalation* may be used every few hours to clear the head, and raising the head end of the bed some four to six inches at night will lessen nasal congestion without the risk of a stiff neck from the use of many pillows. The old idea of 'feeding a cold' lessens congestion in the head temporarily by diverting the circulation to the digestive organs.

Aspirin or *paracetamol*, two tablets three or four times in 24 hours for an adult, will relieve muscular pain and headache. If head or face ache is severe and worse on waking, or when the head is hung down, suspect *sinusitis*.

At present, no vaccine is known to protect against attack, and antibiotics at present available are ineffective, though they may be needed in the later stages, if bacterial infection settles in parts already weakened by the cold virus.

It has recently been suggested that cold virus is spread from the nostrils by the fingers, rather than by sneezing. This has some obvious implications for prevention.

Concussion. Results from shaking of the brain inside the skull, caused by a blow or fall. There is usually unconsciousness, lasting from a few seconds to many days. In the latter case, the patient will come under medical care from the beginning, and it is a safe rule that an ambulance or doctor should be called to anyone unconscious. A mild case may come round a few seconds or minutes after an accident, or may be brought home with a history of having been unconscious for a short time after a fall, with no clear memory of events *before* an accident. He may be unwilling to seek medical aid. It is unwise to agree to this, for consider:

1 He may have damaged a blood vessel in the brain which will slowly bleed during the next few hours, causing unconsciousness and eventually death if untreated.
2 Concussion may have been severe enough to leave him a prey to chronic headache or epilepsy if not treated.
3 The fall may have been caused by some illness, such as a *stroke* or *fit* which produced unconsciousness rather than the other way round.

On finding an unconscious patient, and while awaiting expert help, disturb as little as possible:

1 Make sure he is able to breathe and that mouth is not blocked by dentures, vomit, or clotted blood. Clear the mouth with the forefinger if necessary but to make sure vomit or saliva are not inhaled into the breathing tubes, turn patient so that head is sideways, mouth tilted downwards, as described in *Unconsciousness*, making sure that the head, shoulder and hip are all turned in one piece.

If there is any reason to suspect fractured spine (see *Injury, spine*) turning must only be attempted if blood, secretions, or vomit threaten to choke the patient.

2 Provided the surroundings are safe, do not move patient, but cover him with blankets or rugs to maintain warmth, tucking them under him as much as can be done without moving him.

There is no virtue in trying to keep awake a patient who has been concussed. He should be allowed to sleep, but every hour for twelve hours he should be roused sufficiently to understand and reply to a simple question. If the patient cannot be wakened, or becomes increasingly difficult to rouse, the situation is urgent and expert help is needed (UU).

However well he feels, a patient who has been knocked unconscious should not resume work or drive until he has had medical advice. It is now recognized that even mild concussion affects a patient's efficiency and sense of well-being, and that recovery from this may take a few weeks. (see also *Unconsciousness*.)

Constipation. Infrequent or difficult passage of hard motions. Usually due to faulty habits — see *Aperients*. Failure to pass both motion and wind from the bowel for several days may be more than constipation, and medical advice should be sought (S), or (D) if combined with vomiting or spasmodic abdominal pain. Medical advice should also be sought if there is a sudden and maintained change in a previously established bowel habit; and if constipation and diarrhoea occur alternately (C).

Interruption of routine, with reduced fluid intake, as when travelling, may lead to accumulation of hard motion in the rectum. It may be possible to pass this an hour or so after inserting a moistened glycerin suppository, but a Dulcolax suppository has a more positive action. To insert a suppository, first remove its wrapper, lubricate with Vaseline or soapy water, guide it through the anus, then gently push it in with the finger until the suppository is felt to be grasped by the muscle and pulled away from the finger, which may then be removed and cleansed. As a refinement, the finger can be protected by a disposable fingercot, obtainable from the chemist for a few pence.

Constipation in the elderly can be troublesome in several ways. Weakened muscles make the bowel's action less efficient, and in a few days a mass of unpassed motion can accumulate, blocking the bowel but allowing frequent passage of small amounts of liquefied matter by ball-valve action. The patient often believes he has diarrhoea, until an examination by a doctor or nurse reveals the true state of affairs, and leads to proper treatment. A diet lacking the residues found in bran, whole-meal bread, vegetables, and fruit, and a reduction of water intake to avoid frequent urination can also lead to constipation.

Some old people become obsessed with the need for a daily action, do not always remember whether they have had one or not, and worry accordingly. They can be helped by a return to the childhood device of 'ticking off' each day on a calendar. Easy access to a warm, safe lavatory is most important.

Contemplation. One of the lost arts of Western civilization, now needed more than ever before. In contemporary life many citizens of ordinary standing are required to exert powers of decision and action which formerly were only needed by a small governing class; and we have forgotten that the human mind loses its sense of balance if used without regular times for composure, during which the individual rehearses the basic beliefs on which his judgement depends. When religious beliefs were widely held, the daily and weekly acts of worship offered biological advantages, quite apart from any theological consideration. One requires a daily period of ten to twenty minutes, alone and free from fear of interruption, preferably at a fixed time. One may sit, lie, kneel, or sit tailor-wise, and should always assume the same *posture* once trial has found it the best, as one object of the exercise is to bring the mind back daily to a familiar anchorage. Most people start a period of contemplation by reciting a few basic beliefs (or, if they think they lack these, the Lord's Prayer) to themselves, and then allowing their thoughts to come as they will, following each line of thought until another takes its place. At first the practical happenings and problems of the day jostle each other for attention, bringing their loads of emotion, regret, anxiety, and pleasure, and it helps to have spent a few moments reminding oneself of the principles which ought to have guided one, whether or not they did so.

As one becomes more practised, practical matters occupy less of the contemplative period, partly because they are seen to be less important than had been thought, and partly because the tranquillity achieved by contemplation allows the day's work to be done with much less unfinished emotional business.

When one is practised both in contemplation and *relaxation* it may be possible to combine the two, but at first an attempt to do so may make relaxation difficult owing to the tensions produced by the free flow of thought.

Contraception. This is a subject for individual advice from your doctor. If he is not himself expert, he can introduce you to a Family Planning Clinic. These Clinics (now part of the National Health Service) used to deal mostly with women, but husband-and-wife consultations are increasing, particularly since the availability of vasectomy.

Two points about oral contraceptives ('the Pill') may be mentioned here:

1 Women taking the Pill should be familiar with the early signs of *thrombosis* so that they know what to do should they develop this uncommon complication.
2 Even a short attack of diarrhoea or vomiting, or both, can endanger the contraceptive effect of the Pill. Anyone suffering an attack should take additional precautions for the rest of the cycle, if necessary asking advice from doctor or Family Planning Clinic.

Convulsion. An alarming childhood disturbance. The whole body becomes rigid, the arms held stiffly out with clenched fingers, the eyes open and staring or sometimes rolled upward. The breath is held, the face becomes blue or later white, and foam may appear at the mouth. After a few minutes the stiffness is followed by a convulsive shaking of the limbs and trunk, after which the child relaxes and may fall asleep. The bowel or bladder may empty themselves in the course of the attack. The doctor should be sent for (**U** or **UU**) though only in the rarest and most severe cases will the attack still be in progress when he arrives, and the treatment of a convulsion must be carried out by those present when it starts.

First, understand that three quarters of the attacks end in the course of a few minutes, however long these may seem at the time. Tilt the child so that its head is the lowest part, and turn him so that the mouth is downward. In this position any food which has been returned from the stomach will fall from the mouth, and neither it nor saliva will be inhaled when he finally takes a breath. This head-down position also helps to maintain the circulation in the brain — important in the rare case in which the rigid stage lasts a long time.

Convulsions usually occur in younger children who do not normally have any dental corrective apparatus in their mouths. If they are known to have such, it should be removed early in the attack. After the convulsive movements are over, the child is kept comfortably lying in a normal sleeping position until the doctor sees him.

The commonest cause of convulsion is the rapidly rising temperature at the onset of an illness such as tonsillitis, measles, or pneumonia, and unless the child is quite certainly not feverish, treatment with tepid sponging (described under *Delirium*) should be started as soon as the convulsion is over.

After a convulsion, a child will usually be ordered treatment to be taken either continually or when colds or other illnesses threaten. It is important to follow instructions closely. (See p. 93.)

Breath-holding attacks may be confused with convulsions. In these, the child has a habit of holding his breath when crossed or upset, and continues to do so until he produces a convulsion. If it is recognized as a breath-holding attack from the start, the prompt application of a cold sponge to the back of the neck and between the shoulders may cut it short. This treatment should be applied without any display of emotion and with as little appearance of alarm as possible. The attacks usually indicate the need for an overhaul in the management of the child, and the doctor should be consulted (C).

Corns. Hard patches on toes or soles which may be painful. Usually caused by pressure of ill-fitting shoes. May be confused with verrucas, which are *warts* growing into the thickness of the non-hairy skin.

Treatment: Soaking for ten minutes in comfortably hot *isotonic saline* each night. Nothing else should be attempted unless advised by chiropodist or doctor (C). Do not try to cut or shave them. Ask the cobbler to ease the shoe, or treat it as described under *Bunion*.

Coronary Attack (Coronary Occlusion, Coronary Thrombosis). Blockage of a coronary artery by clotted blood or a fragment from its lining. The heart is a bag-shaped pump made of muscle. With each heartbeat, the muscle contracts, squeezing blood round the circulation. The energy requirements of the heart muscles are met by the coronary arteries, which branch through them, carrying oxygen and fuel in the blood they contain. If a branch of a coronary artery is blocked, its segment of muscle is deprived of blood and not only can it not work, but in the absence of oxygen it dies. If the blockage is in a small artery, the amount of muscle affected may be so small that the patient is not aware of any discomfort or ill-effect, and many of us have had several small coronary occlusions, and have recovered from them, without knowing. Of course, such minor incidents are not what is usually understood by the phrase 'having a coronary', and in a severe attack, a wedge of muscle occupying the whole thickness of the heart wall is temporarily put out of action. If strain is put on it, it may give way, with fatal results; apart from that, the loss of its working ability will deprive the heartbeat of part of

- If a patient is not within the scope of home care, or worsens in spite of it, or if there is any uncertainty, a doctor should be consulted.

its efficiency. If this loss is too high, circulation to vital organs will be impaired.

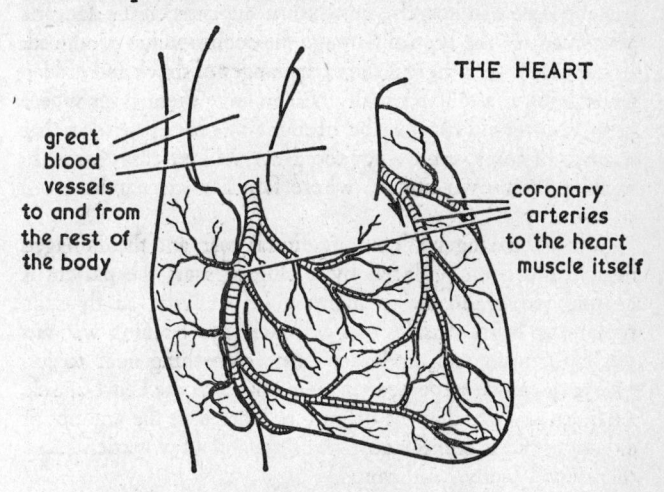

THE HEART

great blood vessels to and from the rest of the body

coronary arteries to the heart muscle itself

The first sign of a coronary occlusion is usually pain of rapid or sudden onset, most often felt in the centre of the chest, sometimes centrally just below the rib cage. The pain often spreads up to the neck, jaws, and one or both shoulders and arms, and varies from moderate to very severe. In a severe attack, the patient is pale, with cold flabby skin, and may vomit. Pain can start either at rest or during exercise, and can be mistaken at first for *angina*, if the patient is familiar with that. However, this is not relieved by trinitrate or amyl nitrite, and these should not be used (or if used at the start of an attack, should not be repeated when found ineffective).

As no home remedy will avail, the doctor should at once be given an idea of the severity of the attack, so that he can judge how urgent the case is. *Keep the patient at rest* in bed or in a comfortable chair until the doctor sees him, with a guarded *hot water bottle* at his feet, and warmly wrapped. If vomiting, try sips of soda water. Spirits should not be given. If he becomes breathless, support him in a sitting position with pillow or a *back-rest*.

Treatment aims at reducing the work the heart has to do by

resting the patient and relieving pain and anxiety, to allow time for repair of the damaged area. Whether or not the patient is best in hospital or at home depends on his doctor's assessment of the type of damage the occlusion has produced. In a severe attack there is the early danger of shock and sudden heart failure, and it is usually best to have these cases where prompt intervention can be brought to bear, provided that hazards of transport are not too great. Milder cases often do well in their own homes, where familiar surroundings aid tranquillity.

When the danger of complication is past, and the damaged muscle has been replaced by a plug of scar, the patient is encouraged gradually to increase his activity, so that the remaining heart muscles can get back into training without strain. In mild and moderate cases, something near to full recovery can be expected. If the damage to the heart muscle has been severe, there is often a reduction in the amount of exertion that is comfortable and safe; and a few patients find themselves badly handicapped.

Once convalescence is over, in the absence of other advice, it is usually safe to undertake exertion which does not make one short of breath and which does not produce central chest pain. The post-coronary patient is in real danger of restricting his activity too much from an unnecessary fear of harming himself. The knowledge that he has had a HEART ATTACK, which most of us spell to ourselves in capital letters, increases anxiety. He should recognize that most of the happenings attributed to his heart are really in his head, and re-read the second sentence of this section to de-glamorize this necessary, prosaic, and hard-working organ.

It is now widely believed that cigarette smoking, obesity, lack of exercise, excessive consumption of fats of animal origin and refined sugar, play a part in producing the 'furring up' of the coronary arteries which favours occlusion. Recent work suggests that older women of child-bearing age run an increased risk of coronary disease while taking an oral contraceptive.

Cough. A cough occurs when something irritates the lining of the breathing passages (except in the nose, where a sneeze serves the same purpose). Unless it achieves the removal of unwanted material — phlegm, or inhaled foreign matter — it is useless and exhausting, and should if possible be prevented. From above downwards the sites in which inflammation can give rise to short term cough are as follows:

Vocal Cords (at the top of the windpipe). Seldom causes cough in the adult; usually loss of voice. In the younger child can cause the sudden onset of croup, in which the child awakes frightened with a short barking brassy cough and defective voice. Occasionally croup may be so severe as to interfere with breathing and help is then needed (UU). More often, the attack will be relieved after sipping a hot sweet drink, and spending twenty or thirty minutes in a warm kitchen or bathroom, in which a kettle and one or two saucepans are kept boiling. The patient can then be returned to bed in a warm room in which two or three washing-up bowls of hot water

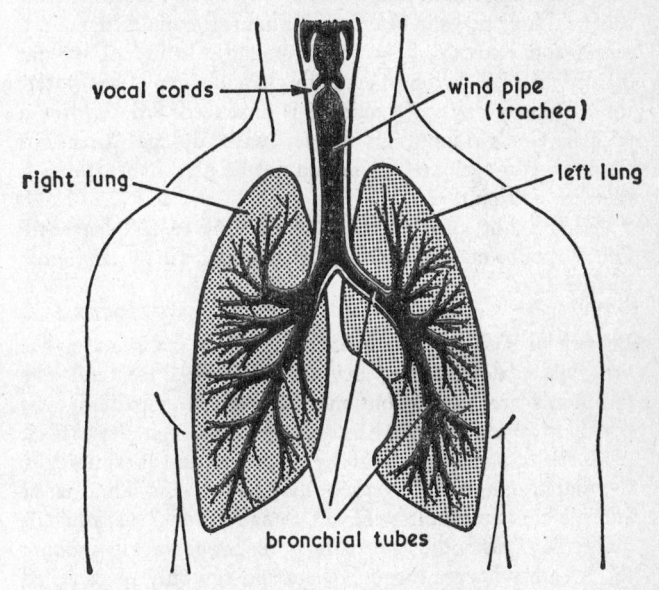

The lungs and breathing passages

are exposed, to moisten the air. Croup in infants may be severe and should be seen by a doctor (D or U, exceptionally UU).

Windpipe (tracheitis). the commonest cause of cough; the ordinary cough which follows a common cold and lasts for five to ten days, harsh and dry at first, later producing more or less phlegm which may be white, yellow, or greyish. If it is green, consult the doctor, as an antibiotic may be needed (S or C).

Uncomplicated tracheitis has traditionally been treated with cough mixtures and linctuses. The cry is increasingly heard that the money spent by the N.H.S. on these should be used for more urgent matters, there being no scientific proof that they do good. The first is undoubtedly true. As to the second, many sufferers claim that their experience tells them otherwise. Such independent spirits will no doubt continue to ease discomfort with *paracetamol* or buy Gee's Linctus, a 5 ml spoonful four times in twenty-four hours for adults, in the dry stage; and *blackcurrant tea* or compound mixture of sodium chloride B.N.F. two 5 ml spoonfuls in half a cup of hot water, three times a day once phlegm is produced. For children a special Gee's Linctus is made, with dosage directions according to age. Linctus should not be used if breathing is rapid or difficult.

A hard, hot, dry cough with fever up to 103 degrees F (39.5°C) or so may be the only sign of measles in the first three to five days.

Bronchial Tubes (acute bronchitis). Here, the infection has progressed downwards beyond the windpipe and the symptoms are similar but more severe. The patient feels poorly in general and may be drowsy. The cough, dry at first, gives rise to pain felt behind the chest bone and as far down as the diaphragm, and the patient may be feverish. Children of allergic constitution may have asthmatic bronchitis, which is marked by spasmodic narrowing of the bronchial tubes so that the breath wheezes through them and can only be expelled with difficulty. The doctor is needed (D) and meanwhile treatment as for croup. Do not give Gee's Linctus. If severe (U), or very occasionally (UU).

Treatment for acute bronchitis: As for tracheitis in the early stages, but the doctor's help is usually necessary, and always so for children or old or frail people. Do not delay because the patient seems better in the morning. If he has had a bad night, let the doctor know in the morning; otherwise he will have to make a late call when the patient worsens in the evening, as is usual, and another night will be sacrificed because a day's treatment has been lost.

In bronchopneumonia, the infection has reached a stage further and infected the lungs, the symptoms are much more severe and the obvious illness of the patient shows that medical care is needed (D).

In lobar pneumonia there is usually no preceding cold or catarrh and the picture is of the sudden onset of a severe feverish illness in which cough plays a part. There may be pain in the chest, worse on coughing, or such pain may be felt in the abdomen or a shoulder. The patient may shiver uncontrollably as the temperature rises, and in children there may be vomiting or a *convulsion* at the onset. In any case, the patient is obviously ill and the doctor is needed (D). Meanwhile, frequent hot drinks, *steam inhalations* and *aspirin* or *paracetamol* will give some relief.

Chronic (Long-term) Cough. A cough should not be allowed to continue for more than two or three weeks without medical advice. In adults, the commonest cause of chronic cough is chronic *bronchitis*. Other causes include tuberculosis, lung cancer, and bronchiectasis. See the doctor (C). In children, cough lasting more than two or three weeks is usually *whooping cough*. The characteristic whoop on the intake of breath after a spasm of coughing usually starts in the second of third week; even without it, a cough which leaves the child red in the face after a spasm, and perhaps leads to vomiting, is suspicious (V).

Cramp. A painful spasm in a muscle, usually of the leg, of which the cause is not known. The limb should be placed so that the cramped muscle is stretched, the muscle then being grasped and squeezed firmly until cramp abates. Avoid cold sheets and tightly made beds. Allow free movement for the feet at the foot of the bed. Severe and recurrent cramp can often be helped by taking quinine, but for this a doctor should be consulted (S). Cramp while swimming causes many drownings, both of victims and would-be rescuers. Nobody subject to cramp should venture out of his depth unless within a few strokes of a manned raft. A swimmer who has never had cramp should ask himself what will happen should he have his first attack while carrying out a projected swim, acting on the assumption that *you cannot have cramp and swim at the same time*, although you can, and should, keep yourself afloat by using the unaffected limbs.

The term is sometimes applied to two important conditions which are not cramp:

1 A patient who has been in bed for over a week, who then gets up and complains of 'cramp' in one or both calves when he walks should return to bed and stay there until his doctor has been able to assure himself that he has not developed *thrombosis* in a vein (D).
2 'Cramp' coming on in the calf after walking a certain distance, which disappears when the patient stands still, reappearing after a further amount of walking, is probably 'intermittent claudication' due to slowing of the circulation to the leg muscles. Consult the doctor (S).

Croup (see *Cough*).

Cuts. A flesh cut should be washed under running cold water for a few minutes, gently dried, then covered with a dry *dressing*. If the skin edges fall together naturally, and the knife was a clean one, daily dry dressing is continued until healing occurs. If the edges gape or there is a risk that the cut was contaminated with earth or infected material, it should be shown to a doctor the same day — as also if there is a possibility of damage to a tendon ('leader') or nerve, shown by inability to make some of the normal movements of the affected part or loss of sensation in any part of the skin. See also *Bleeding* and *Wounds*.

Cyst. A smooth bag of fluid caused by obstruction to the outflow of a *gland*. The commonest are sebaceous cysts of the skin, varying in size from a pea to a walnut, and frequent on the scalp, where they interfere with the care of the hair. If one is accidentally injured by a comb it may burst, expelling its unpleasant smelling contents. The cyst then collapses, giving rise to the hope that it has disappeared, which is disappointed when it refills. (See illustration, p. 218).

Occasionally, a sebaceous cyst becomes inflamed and painful, and should be shown to the doctor (S). It will be eased by hot packs or *hot bathing* while waiting. The removal of sebaceous cysts is a minor surgical operation. There are many other forms of cyst, internal and external, but their nature is not easily apparent and they are subjects for medical diagnosis. (See *Stye*.)

Cystitits. Inflammation of the bladder resulting in a burning pain felt on passing water, or just afterwards. There may be blood in the urine at the onset. Keep an ounce or so and take it to the doctor in a bottle (S). Meanwhile, take a level teaspoonful of bicarbonate of soda three times in the day (for one day only), and drink plenty of water. (See also under *Pain* on passing water, and U and I.)

Dandruff. A common infection of the scalp. It consists of numerous small scales which scatter when the hair is brushed and can then be seen on the clothing and in the brush. The use of an infected brush can spread the disease. It is often combined with a greasy skin and scalp, and the scales falling on the face and shoulders can contribute to *acne* and 'seborrhoeic eczema'. Eczema of the scalp in infants can often be traced to dandruff in one of the family.

Dandruff is often at its worst during adolescence, as is *acne*. It can usually be controlled by washing the scalp two or three times a week in a warm 1 per cent solution of centrimide. Buy a 20 per cent solution and make up one tablespoonful to half a pint with hot water. (Or two 5 ml spoonfuls to 200 ml.) Rub well into the scalp then rinse clear with warm water. Once under control, the cetrimide can be used less often — weekly or fortnightly. If this treatment is not effective, consult the doctor (C).

To prevent re-infection the hair brushes and comb should be washed daily and pillowslips changed daily, being boiled each time, until control is established. If acne is present, the daily changing and boiling should be extended to face cloths, towel, and vest; the latter preferably of cotton.

Deafness. The only form of deafness in which home treatment plays a part is that caused by wax in the ear passage (see illustration, p. 40). Wax is a natural protective secretion which usually falls out of its own accord. Dusty work, a narrow ear passage, or too vigorous a toilet, such as the poking in of towel corners, may delay this, and the compressed wax may swell in damp weather or after bathing, causing sudden loss of hearing. Provided there has been no previous ear disease, the wax can be softened by letting six or eight drops of glycerin, olive oil or nut oil soak into the ear for ten minutes at a time, two or three times before going to the doctor. Removal will then be quicker and more comfortable.

All other forms of deafness need professional advice (C).

The Royal National Institute for the Deaf, 105 Gower Street, London, WC1E 6AH, offers free and confidential help for 'any problem whatever connected with hearing'.

Deafness in Children: As with *squint*, the sooner it is recognized, the better. Even in the first three months, a baby is startled by a loud sound, and deafness may be suspected as early as this by failure to notice a door slamming (but loud sounds should not be used deliberately for testing). From 1 to 3 months, most sounds are unfamiliar to a baby, and if he hears one, such as a voice or rattle, he will stop any activity he is engaged in. At 4 to 5 months, some sounds have become familiar, and on hearing them — mother's voice, his own rattle, etc he turns his eyes in the sound's direction. At 8 months, a baby will turn and look at the source of a familiar sound, and his own voice begins to mimic the rise and fall of normal speech. (At 6 to 8 months a child may not be startled by loud sounds as he has been earlier. This is normal and does not indicate deafness.) Delay in reaching the stages mentioned above should prompt consultation with one's doctor, who may advise a specialist's opinion. Should it prove that there is some deafness, the use of a hearing aid may be advised. This often comes as a shock to parents, who see it as a defeatist measure; but once they understand that the development of *speech* depends on *hearing*, they are glad to co-operate. The earlier a child's brain becomes aware of the sound of speech, the sooner will he start to speak himself. A normal child hears voices for a year or so from birth before starting to make words, and it must be expected that a deaf child will need to use a hearing aid for at least as long before speech begins.

Advice, support and help may be had from the National Deaf Children's Society, 45 Hereford Road, Bayswater, London, W2 5AH.

Death. Is the patient alive and unconscious, or recently dead? Breathing cannot be discerned and the pulse cannot be felt at the wrist. If alive, it should be possible to hear the heartbeat by placing the ear on the skin below the left breast. Open the eyelids and look at the eyes. Within a few minutes of death, the pupils are wide open, the coloured part of the eye has shrunk to a narrow band. As time passes, a blue mottling, like bruising, appears in those parts of the skin lying lowest, the brow is perceptibly cool to the hand and the earliest stage of rigor mortis stiffens the jaw, so that the mouth cannot be opened or shut. If in doubt, proceed as for *unconsciousness*.

Delirium. A confused state of semi-consciousness in which the patient, under the influence of illness, has visual impressions of monsters, animals, etc, sometimes based on the shapes of shadows or patterns of decoration. Often experienced by children with high temperatures in the course of acute illnesses, such as measles. Gentle reassurance, sponging with luke-warm water from head to foot, then dry towelling, will usually allow natural sleep, though the sponging may need to be repeated once or twice. Acute illness in an elderly patient, such as *pyelitis* or *pneumonia*, can produce a confusional state. It is unwise to sponge these patients without expert advice, but a *cold pack* to the brow, frequently renewed, may help. Delirium can be produced by alcoholic poisoning (delirium tremens), and should be suspected when a heavy drinker suddenly shows a distaste for alcohol, is sleepless, and seems to be in fear; also when a heavy drinker confined to bed by illness makes scrabbling movements at the bedding 'like a puppet leaning out of a window', or makes remarks which are out of key with the actual circumstances. Any delirious adult who seems in danger of harming himself or others needs medical care promptly (UU).

Depression. The name of a group of mental illnesses in which the main symptom is usually what would in everyday terms be called depression. Some people have a constitutional tendency to attacks, sometimes alternating with periods of excitement and increased or exaggerated activity of mind and body. When these last occur, they serve the purpose of putting those around the patient on their guard against the following attack of depression. Without this warning and in those non-recurring attacks of depression produced by the stress of work or worry, illness, adolescence or menopause, and sometimes before or after childbirth, the onset of depressive illness may be suspected by a change of mood, poor sleep (particularly waking in the early hours), inability to get going in the morning, slowness to reply to questions, as though thinking of something else, and sometimes a demeanour of fatigue and distress, though a person of strong character may consciously conceal the last.

The recognition of depression in a patient by those around him is of importance, as early treatment diminishes the risk of suicide to which some depressives are exposed. Every effort should be made to persuade the patient to seek medical help, and if he refuses, in severe cases or those in which there is a sharp worsening of the condition, or when the patient mentions the possibility of suicide, those concerned should themselves get in touch with the patient's doctor, the same day.

Above all, *never advise the patient to 'pull himself together'*. He would if he could, but he is no more able to than a man with a broken leg is to walk.

Dermatitis. Roughly equivalent to *eczema*.

Dhobie Itch. A fungus infection of the groin. (See under *Ringworm*).

Diabetes Mellitus. The patient's pancreas gland (see illustration, p. 155) does not produce enough insulin to make proper use of the carbohydrates (sugar and starch) which he eats. The sugar is lost in the urine and abnormal waste products accumulate in the patient's system, leading eventually to diabetic coma. Diabetes may be suspected when a patient who has lost weight and complains of thirst and passing a lot of urine becomes drowsy and finally unconscious, although he will usually have attracted medical attention long before the latter.

Many diabetics need to use insulin injections daily and to regulate their diet so that they take enough carbohydrate to provide fuel for the body's work, and enough insulin to put it to use. These quantities will be advised by the doctor or diabetic clinic they attend regularly. They will be taught to check the urine they pass for detection of unused sugar and to seek advice if this becomes excessive. Insulin requirements go up at times of illness, and the doctor should be informed of any but trivial illnesses, in case an increased dose of insulin is indicated. Illnesses involving vomiting are particularly difficult to treat, as the patient may not be able to keep down enough carbohydrate to use up his injection of insulin. The result is a reduction in the amount of sugar in the blood below that needed for the proper working of the brain, and this can lead to confusional behaviour resembling drunkenness, and to unconsciousness — 'hypoglycaemic coma', which has to be distinguished from diabetic coma and treated accordingly. Hypoglycaemic coma can occur from a reduction of carbohydrate intake for any reason, such as delay in feeding while travelling, or from unusual physical activity, and all diabetics are advised to carry sugar with them so that they can swallow some quickly if they feel an attack threatening. A known diabetic who is found to be drowsy and/or confused should be persuaded to swallow three or four sugar lumps or three teaspoonfuls of sugar or glucose, with a drink. *No attempt should be made to administer sugar or water to an unconscious patient.* The dose of sugar should be repeated after about fifteen minutes, and medical advice sought, unless the patient is known to be familiar with the management of attacks, and will not be alone overnight. Coma — *unconsciousness* from whatever cause — is an emergency and requires urgent medical care (UU) or admission to hospital by ambulance.

Diabetics are liable to foot trouble and should be encouraged to take greater care of their feet than others. Daily washing and changing of socks, well-fitting socks and shoes, weekly trimming of the nails, and early medical attention to any sort of injury on the foot will help to avoid trouble which can be difficult to halt, once started.

For milder diabetes, usually in older people, treatment by mouth can sometimes take the place of insulin injections. Attention to accurate dosage and diet and regular checks at the doctor's or clinic is just as important as when insulin is used.

All diabetics should consider joining the British Diabetic Association, 10 Queen Anne St, London, W1M 0BD, which publishes a journal for diabetics, among other services.
Note: Hypoglycaemic attacks in children can be mistaken for naughtiness or 'playing up', and any alteration in a diabetic child's usual behaviour pattern should alert his family. Severe attacks can cause *convulsions*.

Diarrhoea. Frequent and often painful passage of loose or liquid motions from the bowel. The commonest cause is acute enteritis (see *Gastroenteritis* for treatment), caused by inflammation of the intestine by a *germ* or by contaminated food. This usually lasts for hours rather than days, and is covered under *Gastroenteritis*.

Diarrhoea lasting for several days or weeks should be medically investigated: so should alternating attacks of diarrhoea and constipation, and diarrhoea with passage of blood (S or V).

Soreness of the anus following a sharp attack of diarrhoea will be eased by the application of *hot packs* once or twice.

See also *Kaolin Mixture*, *Dysentery*, and the chapter *Newborn*.

Diet. For home treatment purposes it may be taken that, unless a particular diet is mentioned for any condition, the patient may be offered a little of what he fancies at fairly frequent intervals (1–3 hours) and that if he does not wish to take food he should not be pressed, but allowed to take a variety of liquids (again, little and often) for a day or two. A few black grapes, a strip of smoked salmon, ice-cream, 'apple snow', or zabaglione, make a welcome addition to the usual invalid fare of soups, cereals, milk puddings, and jellies, and those who like yoghourt should be encouraged to take it.

It is increasingly believed that the average western European diet contains too much refined sugar and animal fat, and too little vegetable roughage, particularly bran; and that this distortion, combined with insufficient exercise, lays the foundation for some of the diseases of middle and old age.

Dieting to reduce weight: see *Obesity*.

Disability. The voluntary and official services which care for and help the disabled are being expanded as funds become available. Social Services Departments are able to arrange for provision of aids, for alteration to the patient's home to allow free passage for a wheelchair, fitting of handrails, etc, and to advise about financial help.

A description of the financial and other help available to the disabled will be found in *The Disability Rights Handbook*, obtainable from The Disability Alliance, 1 Cambridge Terrace, London, NW1. See also The Design Centre's *Handicapped at Home* by Sidney Foott.

The Directory for the Disabled, by Ann Darnborough and Derek Kinrade, published by Woodhead-Faulkner Ltd, 8 Market Passage, Cambridge, CB2 3PF, is a handbook of information and opportunities for disabled and handicapped people.

The Royal Association for Disability and Rehabilitation, 25 Mortimer Street, London, W1N 8AB publishes *Holidays for the Physically Handicapped*. The Automobile Association has a list of hotels for the disabled under the title *Guide for the Disabled* for the use of its members.

Many people wish that they knew how much help, and of what kind, to offer to the disabled. For the blind, the pamphlet *How to Guide a Blind Person* is available from The Royal National Institute for the Blind, 224 Great Portland Street, London, W1N 6AA.

For the deaf, a pamphlet, *Sound Advice: How You Can Help Deaf People*, is issued by the Health Education Council, 78 New Oxford Street, London, WC1A 1AH, and may be available from local health departments or clinics.

Roger Sydenham, of the Royal National Institute for the Deaf, quotes Jonathan Miller, asking "Why are the blind sacred, and the deaf absurd?" Could the difference in attitude towards the two handicaps arise because the blind declare themselves openly, enlisting consideration or help, whereas many deaf people are reluctant to reveal their disability? This often gets the relationship with a deaf person off to a bad start, as he is discovered to be deaf only when he responds in a way which, were he not handicapped, would appear discourteous or stupid. I think the time may have come for anyone handicapped by deafness to identify himself, perhaps by wearing a badge (as is done in parts of Europe), or a thin armband, which could be seen from behind.

The R.N.I.D. are introducing a symbol indicating that the needs of the hard of hearing are recognized, for use at information desks, etc, which, when sufficiently well recognized, might serve as a personal badge. They tell me that the take-up of personal badges indicating deafness was so low that they are no longer supplied. As I suggest above, I think sufferers should re-consider their unwillingness to be identified. There is a store of goodwill waiting to be tapped.

Disc, Slipped. A convenient but sometimes inaccurate description of the painful locking of one of the spinal joints. (See *Lumbago* and *Spondylosis*.)

Discharge, Vaginal. The vagina is a moist cavity, as is the nose, and in both some of the natural mucus sometimes escapes to the outside. Although this natural secretion is not usually noticeable, it can at times amount to a nuisance when the lower abdominal organs are congested, around the time of menstruation. Remedial measures should include gentle daily cleansing with warm soapy water — the increasing use of bidets in this country should help to enable this to be done. Shaving the pubic hair prevents retention of the secretion on the skin. Scented toilet water applied externally is useful, but the use of lotions with a chemical smell serves more to draw attention than divert it. Internal applications are not advised unless on medical advice, as they disturb the balance of the vaginal fluids. The same applies to the use of a douche. Any discharge which exceeds the degree mentioned, is offensive, or gives rise to irritation of the skin should be medically investigated (S).

Dislocation. Occurs when, as a result of violence, the two bones making up a joint are forced out of their usual relationship. Thus in a ball-and-socket joint, such as the shoulder, the ball on the upper end of the arm bone can be forced right out of the shoulder socket to lie above, below, or to the side of it. The powerful muscles attached to the upper arm go into spasm, as a result of the pain caused, and it is not usually justifiable to try to correct such a dislocation without an X-ray and anaesthetic. The forearm is supported by a sling (see illustration, p. 151), the upper arm held against the chest with a scarf or bandage to prevent painful movement, and the patient taken to hospital. It will not be possible to give an anaesthetic for four hours after food or drink has been taken, so this should be avoided unless a long journey is entailed, when half a cup of water or tea could be given every half hour, or more often if thirst is complained of.

Dislocation of the end-bone of a finger or thumb sometimes occurs on the sports field, and in the first few seconds afterwards a resolute friend sometimes takes advantage of the numbness to give a good pull to the displaced section, which when released may resume its normal position. If the patient has not benefited from such a happy combination of chance and good intent, he should take himself to hospital or doctor within a few hours.

Another athletic dislocation is that of the knee-cap. On comparison with the other knee, it can be seen that the knee-cap is lying to the side of the joint — not always easy to recognize, as the swelling which occurs quickly confuses the appearance. It needs hospital treatment.

Dog Bite. Victims of dog bite were once sent to their doctors for cauterization of the wound. This painful manoeuvre was practised for the prevention of rabies (hydrophobia) in the nineteenth century.

The United Kingdom is free from rabies, and may well remain so unless someone asserts their independence by smuggling an infected pet from the Continent. Outside this country, a dog bite, however small, should always have early medical attention (S or D — see *Rabies*).

A much more active risk is that the dog has recently been admiring horse manure or manured earth, so that there is a possibility of tetanus, and a dog bite should be seen by a doctor the same day so that the need for protection can be assessed.

Dressings. The best dressing for damaged skin is plain sterile gauze, held in place by a bandage. This protects the wound from infection by germs and allows the evaporation of excess moisture. Packets of gauze (half, or one metre, or single swabs) can be bought ready sterilized from the chemist, and as their sterility is lost once they are open, it is better to have several small packets than one large one. If the dressing is likely to stick, a single piece of paraffin gauze taken fresh from its tin and trimmed to size, is applied first of all. It is important not to touch or contaminate the suface of the dressing which is to go on the wound. Hands should be washed and dried, and scissors, etc, boiled for five to ten minutes before doing a dressing. For trivial injuries, these precautions are not always observed, and clean gauze or linen is used, or a proprietary first-aid dressing applied. A so-called waterproof dressing should only be kept on while protection from water is needed, for what keeps water out will also keep it in, and a soggy wound or burn encourages the spread of infection. Similarly, if a gauze dressing is fixed by plaster, sufficient gauze should be exposed to the air to allow 'breathing'. In the ordinary way, dressings for small injuries should be changed daily or every other day once healing is advanced — more often only if soaked with discharge or if the part is accidentally wetted. Some redressing can be avoided if the part can be enclosed in a polythene bag while washing or bathing.

In emergencies, laundered sheets or towels, with a preference for those that have been boiled, or the inside sheets of hitherto unopened newspapers have been used. Any cut or injury where the skin edges gape open, where skin or flesh has been lost, or where bone can be seen in, or coming out of, the wound, needs medical care within a few hours — in the latter case after competent first aid for possible fracture. (See also *Burns, Cuts, First Aid, Wounds*.)

Dropsy. An old name given to a form of swelling of the legs — see *Swollen legs*.

Drowning. A way of dying, caused by the entry of water into the lungs. Once the patient has stopped breathing, he has four or five minutes* to live unless competent first aid is at hand. Every parent — some would say every adult — should master a method of *artificial respiration*, preferably mouth-to-mouth, and preferably learnt at a *first-aid* class. The following summary is a reminder, not a substitute for practical instruction.

1 Get patient ashore if it can be done within two minutes. If not, practise mouth-to-mouth respiration *in the water*.
2 Clear mouth and throat of any debris.
3 Bend head well back to open the breathing passages.

* Recently, some remarkable delayed recoveries have been recorded with only minor brain damage, when immersion was in sufficiently cold water to 'refrigerate the brain'. In view of this, if the immersion was in water below 70°F (21°C), as it is around the United Kingdom for most of the year, artificial respiration should be continued for two hours before hope is abandoned.

4 Start artificial respiration. After first few breaths, quickly place ear against skin under the left breast to listen for heartbeat, or feel for a carotid pulse. One lies deep to the front edge of each of the muscles which form a V from below the ears to the breast bone, half way along. If you can hear the heart beat, or feel a pulse, the heart is working. Resume artificial respiration until patient breathes on his own. If not,

5 Perform external heart massage, placing palms of hands over each other on the lowest part of the breast bone and pressing it back towards the spine — extent of movement about an inch — once a second — until the heart starts to beat. Every six to eight seconds give four or five puffs of artificial respiration, or let a third party continue to do that while you do the heart massage. Do not be rough. It is easy to fracture ribs and injure the lungs by excessive zeal. Heart massage can only be done if patient is ashore or aboard, his back firmly supported.

6 Send anyone available for medical help as soon as possible.

7 The chance of recovery from near-drowning is worse in fresh water than sea water, for chemical reasons. There have been conflicting opinions about 'draining the lungs', most holding that it wastes times which should be spent starting artificial respiration. However, it is now advised that after salt water immersion, if possible, a few seconds be spent tipping the patient up by his legs to allow water to drain from the mouth. This reduces later complications.

See also *Cramp* and *Exposure*.

Drug. A word loaded with emotion and double meaning. To the doctor, nearly all the substances which he uses in the treatment of disease are called drugs; for that is the original meaning. In general speech, the term implies dangerous drugs or drugs of addiction, and confusion can arise when a patient tells his doctor that he is unwilling to be treated with 'drugs'. To the doctor, if strictly applied, this would remove a great part of his usefulness to the patient.

In present day medical practice, doctors have available a great range of powerful treatments which did not exist a generation ago. The use of these can bring great advantages in treatment of certain diseases or complaints, but they are ordered for a particular condition in a particular patient, and should be used for no other purpose or person. In some, the effect depends on continued use, and omission can have even more serious results than an overdose. A proportion of patients will find that they cannot tolerate a treatment ordered, by reason of unusual sensitivity, so that it may produce for instance, nausea, giddiness, or undue sleepiness. If that happens, report the trouble to the doctor as soon as possible (S). Alteration of the dose or the treatment may be called for. Sometimes, the treatment may have to be abandoned, and the patient should ask the doctor for a note of the substance, so that he can carry a record of his intolerance of that treatment — see *Medic Alert*. (See also *Addiction to drugs*.)

Duodenal Ulcer. An *ulcer* of the tube which leads partly digested food from the stomach to the intestine (see illustration, p. 155). It is often produced by a combination of anxiety, tension, and irregular feeding in a person constitutionally predisposed.

Although occasionally 'silent', giving rise to no pain, a typical duodenal ulcer causes pain two or three hours after a meal, which is relieved by taking food. Pain may wake the patient in the early morning and be relieved by a few mouthfuls of milk. Diagnosis is by X-ray or gastroscope (C).

The dangers of bleeding and perforation are the same as described under *Gastric ulcer* (UU). (See also *Peptic Ulcer*.) Duodenal ulcer patients should never take *aspirin*.

Dying, Care of the. The successful management of a patient known to be dying requires an alteration in the climate of thought surrounding him. Many of the activities pursued in the hope of recovery are now useless, or worse. The aim is now the maintenance of the patient's comfort for a period of hours or days — nothing beyond. He no longer needs food — may choke if given it; nor drink, beyond the little fluid necessary to keep the mouth from drying. As he may not be able to swallow, any fluid given may go the wrong way into the lungs. The tongue, if dry, can be lightly smeared with vaseline, and a wick of folded gauze run in through the mouth to lie between gums and cheek. A few chips of ice may be enclosed in this, or it may be moistened with drops of water from time to time. If too much saliva is being produced, turn the head so that the corner of the mouth with the wick in it is downwards, to allow drainage.

The kidneys will continue to send urine to the bladder, and if this is not emptied, severe discomfort can arise. A urinal or bedpan should be placed in position every two hours and left for five or ten minutes. A time-sheet of urine passed and roughly the quantity, should be kept, and doctor or nurse can empty the bladder artificially if it becomes distended. No attempt should be made to provoke a bowel action. Packing with cellulose wadding (bought in 500 gram packets) will absorb leakage from bladder or bowel. As far as possible, the bedding should be kept dry and unwrinkled; incontinence pads can usually be provided by the District Nurse.

The patient is often propped up in a half or full sitting position for easier breathing. Remember to support the two spinal hollows, the neck and the small of the back, with suitably placed pillows or cushions.

Keep the room well lit unless the patient wishes otherwise. It should not be overheated. The patient's skin may feel cold but *he* is more likely to feel too hot than too cold. Watch for efforts to throw off the bedding, which may indicate this, and reduce the cover accordingly.

There must always be doubt as to how conscious the dying person is, and it is better to assume that he can feel and comprehend. Let someone sit holding his hand for a while. Speak in ordinary voices and *Never Whisper*. If something must be said which he must not hear, go outside to say it, or write it. (See also *Nursing*.)

Dysentery. A severe continuing diarrhoea. In the U.K. we see only the mild form, Sonne dysentery, and the features typical of tropical dysenteries — passing of blood, prostration, liver damage, are not usual, unless caught abroad (V or D). Some Sonne dysentery is always present in the United Kingdom, probably owing to a reservoir of *carriers*. In an attempt to reduce this, the Community Physician may arrange several stool tests after a patient has recovered. These will show whether a patient has completely eliminated the disease, and indicate the need for further treatment if he has not. It is wise to cooperate in these measures, to avoid the risk of spreading infection to one's family, and beyond. (See *Hygiene, personal*.)

Dyspepsia (See *Indigestion*).

Earache. May accompany tonsillitis or toothache, but is most often due to inflammation behind the ear drums. This may burst through the drum, leading to discharge from the ear. Earache which is not abolished by two or three *aspirin* or *paracetamol* tablets — adult doses — (for children's doses, see under *Aspirin* and *Paracetamol*) needs medical treatment, as does a discharging ear, always. Seek aid as early in the day as possible, so that treatment may have a chance to ensure a comfortable night (D or S according to severity and degree of general upset. A child whose earache has kept him awake should always see the doctor the next morning.) Raising the head end of the bed six or seven inches reduces pain.

After an ear infection, the hearing may be temporarily reduced. If there is any doubt about its recovery after one or two weeks, the doctor should be consulted, as further treatment may be called for, although natural improvement can continue for some months.

Earache in babies is a common cause of crying, as mentioned in the Chapter *Newborn*, and of vomiting with or without diarrhoea. (See also under *Adenoids* and *Tonsils*.)

Eczema. An irritation of the skin, usually in those of allergic (see *Allergy*) constitution. It is *not* infectious and can be produced mechanically (as by rubbing an itching patch), by nervous tension, or by various allergic contacts, such as primula, beans, flour, cement, detergents, etc. Common sensitivities are to nickel in costume jewellery and to nail varnish, arising on the neck from stroking the skin with varnished fingertips (**S** or **C**).

The eczema subject should remember that his skin has less than the usual protection against most irritant substances, and should protect the hands with polythene or thin rubber gloves (preferably with removable cotton linings), when handling detergents, soaps, solvents, etc, and with leather or fabric gloves when doing domestic work or gardening.

Suntan should be achieved cautiously, and gloves worn in winter, when the wind is in the east, and great care should be taken in drying the hands after washing. Once eczema is present, even soap and water should be avoided, cleansing being with *isotonic saline*, nut oil, or liquid *paraffin*.

Eczema on a baby should always be seen by the doctor (**C**). It is sometimes caused by *dandruff* falling from the heads of other members of the household, and occasionally by allergy to cows' milk, but this is rare. *Vaccination* against smallpox should not be performed on eczematous patients, and they should be kept away from anyone recently vaccinated. Exzema tends to be more troublesome in spring and autumn. A patient soon gets to know his complaint and how to manage it, and when he needs his doctor's help — a timely consultation if under stress of work or worry will often forestall an attack. The terms eczema and dermatitis are often used to describe the same condition. First aid treatment is with calamine lotion or zinc cream, unless the doctor has ordered anything else. Avoid heavy ointments and antiseptics.

It is not generally known that a patch of eczema anywhere sensitizes the skin of the whole body; so that applying embrocation to one's knee, or using a rough hand cleanser, can produce secondary eczema of those parts, although the original patch may be on the foot.

Electric Shock. The victim is either burned, or unconscious, or both. Is he still in contact with the current? If so, turn it off. If that cannot be done at once, arrange to remove him with minimum delay, using a non-conducting implement (broadly, something non-metallic and dry) to push or pull him away from it. Small appliances can be moved out of contact by pulling on their insulated flex.

If the patient is unconscious, *artificial respiration* is started immediately, after removing any debris, clotted blood, vomit, or displaced dentures from the patient's mouth and nostrils. It is continued for half an hour before stopping to see if the patient is still alive (see *Death*). After the first few movements of artificial respiration, allow a few seconds to feel or listen for the heartbeat under the left breast. If it is absent, an attempt at external cardiac massage (see under *Drowning*) must be made, breaking off every six seconds to give further artificial respiration. These manoeuvres are much easier if a second helper is available, and he should be despatched to call for an ambulance or similar help as soon as he can be spared, if no other messenger is available. Artificial respiration should be continued for several hours or until the patient is pronounced beyond aid by a doctor. A conscious patient's burns should be treated as described under *Burns and Scalds*.

Enuresis (see *Bedwetting*).

Ephedrine. Obtain as tablets of 30 mg and 15 mg of ephedrine hydrochloride. It is useful treatment for taking early in an attack of *asthma*. It should not be used for anyone who has had recent difficuly in passing water, as it may aggravate that complaint. The recommended dose is one 30 mg tablet for adults and children over six, one 15 mg tablet for children one to five years and half a 15 mg tablet for a child under one year, though for younger children treatment will only be given in the absence of medical advice if the condition appears serious.

Epilepsy. A condition of the brain causing the occurrence of 'fits'. There are two common kinds, for which the old names are still used:

Grand Mal (major epilepsy). The fits are not usually frequent, and there is sometimes only one attack in a whole lifetime. More usually, an attack may happen two or three times a year, and there is a rare and serious condition in which the attacks follow each other in close succession — this is sometimes caused by leaving off regular treatment against advice. Before the typical grand mal attack the victim may have a few seconds of warning; sometimes an indescribable sensation in the upper abdomen, sometimes a feeling in a limb. If so, it can serve two purposes — to get him out of a position of danger, and if in a limb, may allow time to prevent the development of the attack by grasping the limb quickly and firmly well above the part in which the sensation is felt. After the warning, if it happens, there is a sudden loss of consciousness and the victim falls to the ground with all his muscles in spasm, so that breathing is obstructed and the face becomes dark and congested. After half a minute or less, the convulsive stage starts, with shaking and writhing movements of the trunk and limbs, biting the tongue and sometimes emptying the bladder. During either stage, the patient can be turned over by the uncoordinated force of the muscles, so that during the following stage of unconsciousness he may smother if he has turned over in bed, or drown if in his bath. He may remain deeply unconscious for half an hour or so, and then pass into a natural sleep or waken in a state of confusion before going to sleep. After a fit, a patient may carry out actions of which he is not conscious and which may endanger himself or others — so-called automatism. Automatism can also occur without a preliminary fit, or after attacks of:

Petit Mal (minor epilepsy) and can then be of greater importance, as these fits are not followed by unconsciousness or sleep, and a mild attack may even be unnoticed by the patient and those around him. Varying in severity, they consist of transient lapses in consciousness, so short that if the patient falls he immediately picks himself up and continues what he was doing. The fits of petit mal usually happen more frequently than those of grand mal.

The task of a bystander when a major fit occurs is to prevent the patient injuring himself during the spasmodic phase. As soon as possible, try to wedge a rolled-up handkerchief or something similar between the gnashing teeth to spare the tongue while allowing air to get past. Once the patient is quiet he will need protection from cold with blankets, and a cushion or pad for his head. Search can then be made for a bracelet, which may indicate that he is a known epileptic and provide his address (see *Medic Alert*). If the fit is in a public place it is safest to send for an ambulance, unless he recovers quickly and will agree to being accompanied home in a car or taxi. The risk of automatic irresponsible behaviour must be borne in mind when anyone recovers from a fit and declares the intention of continuing his business alone. A fit occurring in the home of someone not previously known to have had one should be controlled as above, the patient being got to bed when possible and the doctor sent for (D or U) so that diagnosis can be established.

It is not usually necessary to send for medical help when a known epileptic has a fit unless some injury calls for it, as the patient and those around him will usually be familiar with the pattern of events. A succession of major fits always needs the doctor's help and he should be informed should a patient be known to have left off his regular treatment.

The object of medical treatment is to prevent the fits, or to reduce them to a minimum, and once treatment has started it should be continued without interruption until there have been no fits for a period of two or three years. After that it may be possible gradually to reduce treatment and finally stop it, all under strict medical supervision. This process may well take a year. While epileptics are encouraged to live as normally as possible, there are some obvious limitations. They should not stand on the edge of a railway platform or pavement, nor follow dangerous hill paths. They should not be put within range of falling against moving machinery and should not drive a motor vehicle or bicycle. (In 1970, new regulations allowed the issue of driving licences to patients who had not had an attack while awake for the previous three years, and to some cases of sleeping epilepsy, provided that their driving is not likely to be a source of danger to the public. This applies to private vehicles only.)

Bathing, in shallow water only, should be in the presence of two strong helpers aware of the patient's disability and capable of lifting him ashore. A bath should only be taken if help is within hearing, and the door should never be locked. Some patients are prone to fits during sleep, and these should train themselves to sleep on a firm mattress with no pillow. If a pillow must be used it should be a small firm one (hard stuffed, like a baby's) and should have a weight hung over the edge of the bed by cords from the two outer corners, which will pull the pillow off the bed if convulsions produce irregular pressure of the head on it.

The family and friends of a known case of petit mal should be alert for dangerous or anti-social behaviour following an unnoticed fit and be prepared to exercise whatever restraint the circumstances demand.

Exposure. Severe chilling of the skin surface leading to lowering of body temperature; a major cause of mountain and hill walking causualities, which are increasing every year. Causes:

1. Lack of preliminary training.
2. Lack of sufficient food and drink.
3. Lack of proper clothing, particularly in thin people.
4. Fatigue.
5. Youth and inexperience.

Bad organization can convert an accident into a fatality by adding exposure to it.

Early signs: Unreasonable behaviour, lethargy, abnormal speech, shivering, falling, and complaint of cramp. Anyone showing any of these needs prompt treatment, aimed at preventing heat loss. Dry wrapping, the outer layer water and wind-proof; rest, sheltered from wind while transport is arranged; warm sweet drinks, if able to swallow. He should be seen by a doctor on arrival at base. Failing that, he should be placed in a hot bath (water at 42-45 degrees C = 107-113 degrees F) with his arms out of the water, until his temperature reaches normal or near it, and then put to bed.

The hot bath treatment should also be used for cases of cold immersion (skating and boating accidents, etc). In this connection, the following advice is given to reduce the effects of immersion overboard:

1. On board, wear as much warm clothing as possible, adding

a layer *as soon as* you feel cold. 50% of body heat is lost from the head.
2 Wear an efficient life jacket.
3 Once in the water, do the *minimum swimming* needed to keep afloat or to reach a raft or other buoyancy.
4 Stay with the boat, raft, or lifebuoy; do not try to swim for the shore. Even a short swim in cold water without additional buoyancy can be fatal.

Eye. The commonest cause of a painful inflamed eye is conjunctivitis ('pink eye' is a form of this). The lids are usually stuck together in the morning and should be bathed with pads of cotton wool wrung out of plain hot water. This is a good treatment for most forms of inflammation of the eye while waiting for medical advice, which should always be sought (S).

Conjunctivitis is an infection, and is easily spread to others, and to the other eye. Frequent hand-washing, burning of swabs, pads, etc, that have touched the eye, and segregation of towels and face cloths, which should be boiled each day, as should (cotton) pillow slips, will limit the spread.

Foreign body: Usually dust or soot blown in, scale or metal from unprotected welding or grinding, stone or brick fragments from building work. Many of these accidents result from neglect of safety precautions. If the mote can be seen on the white of the eye or under the turned lid, attempt to wipe it off with a wisp of clean cotton wool or soft cotton. If it will not come off, or is seen over the pupil or coloured part of the eye, attempt no more, but seek medical aid (S).

A burn of the eye with hot fluid or molten metal is an emergency calling for urgent treatment (UU), as is injury by a corrosive fluid. In the last, immediate copious washing with several jugs or cups of cold or luke-warm water allowed to flow freely across the eye (not dropped from a height), with lids held open, will wash out the corrosive. *Copious* washing is important, as a small volume of water in contact with such substances as quicklime, carbolic, or sulphuric acid could make the situation worse.

Black Eye. An injury not of the eye but of the lids and

tissues around it. Caused by a blow releasing blood among these soft tissues, which swell and may close the eye. Occasionally the force of the blow reaches the eyeball itself and can then cause severe injury to it — particularly detachment of the retina, the sensitive nerve network at the back of the eye. It is safest to ask medical advice to exclude any such possibility (**S**). The risk is greater to sufferers from severe short-sight ('high myopia').

Tired Eyes. This usually means 'tired eyelid muscles', which have been overacting in a tendency to 'screw up'. This can result from sight insufficiently good for the work in hand, and usually calls for an eye test by a doctor or ophthalmic optician. Surprisingly often, the sight is found to be normal and the condition to be the result of nervous tension. Short-term treatment is then by hot padding, as above, for five minutes in the evening and at bedtime. Long term, *relaxation* and tranquillity are required.

A *painful eye* always needs medical advice. The more painful it is and the more suddenly it comes on, the more urgent it is (**S** or **D**, accordingly).

(See also *Glaucoma*.) For illustration of eye see P. 72.

Fainting. A short period of unconsciousness caused by temporary failure of the blood supply to the brain. The patient feels momentary uneasiness, often too short to allow him to seek help, his face turns pale and he falls to the ground. There he may make convulsive movements of the limbs for a few seconds before the colour returns to his face and he regains consciousness, provided he has not given himself concussion by striking his head. He should not be encouraged to sit up at once, but should be made comfortable with cushions and rugs while a search is made to exclude *injury*. If none is found, the patient is rested for ten minutes or so, then sat up in a chair and arrangements made to send him home, or to keep him resting

- **If a patient is not within the scope of home care, or worsens in spite of it, or if there is any uncertainty, a doctor should be consulted.**

several hours. Anyone who has been unconscious should not tend machinery or drive a car for several hours and should not be sent home unescorted unless after a period of a few hours' rest he is seen to be in full control of his faculties. For a faint lasting more than a few minutes, see *Unconsciousness*.

Causes and Prevention. The head is at the top of the high-pressure arterial system supplying blood to the whole body, so any lowering of pressure in the system will be noticed there first. Simple gravity is one of the commonest causes of fainting, the legs filling up with blood after the victim has been standing still for a time, as in a parade or school assembly. At first, the muscle tone in the legs prevents an undue amount of blood accumulating, but when the muscles tire and relax, blood is diverted downwards out of the general circulation. Prevent this happening by frequently clenching the toes, calf and thigh muscles for a few seconds at a time, also tighten the buttocks as if to hold a coin between them. Another common cause is stimulation of the vagus nerve network by pain or an unpleasant sight or sound. This can produce a vasovagal attack, with slowing of the heart rate, so that the blood pressure falls. Some susceptible people develop vasovagal attacks from nervous excitement and various other causes. Anyone who knows he might develop an attack should avail himself of the rather longer warning a vasovagal attack usually gives (often a cold sweat and nausea) to sit with his head on his knees or even lie down. A short period of *relaxation* before undertaking a stressful engagement, such as a public dinner or speech, will prevent many attacks.

A common cause of fainting in older people is tilting the head back to hang out clothes, look at a bird, etc. The movement causes kinking of the blood vessels in channels already narrowed by rheumatism in the neck joints, and the blood supply to the brain is obstructed for long enough to produce a faint. These attacks are prevented by avoiding the movement which causes them.

Repeated 'faints': Some people all their lives tend to faint for comparatively minor reasons. They are aware of their disability and learn to live with it or avoid it. Anyone who starts to faint frequently — say two or three times in a year —

needs a medical overhaul, for the 'faints' might be masking a mild form of *epilepsy* which could be treated successfully (C).

Fever. A rise in body temperature above the 'normal', usually taken as 98.6 degrees F (= 37 degrees C) in the mouth. Underarm temperature may be one degree Fahrenheit lower and rectal temperature one degree higher. The mechanism of production of fever is complicated; it usually indicates that there is infection by *germs* — bacteria or virus — somewhere in the body. The term is also applied to particular illnesses — *scarlet*, *glandular*, *typhoid*, *rheumatic*; in all of which a rise of temperature is a feature. See *Temperature taking*.

Tepid sponging makes a feverish patient more comfortable. It is described under *Delirium*.

Fibroids. Lumps of fibrous matter which form in the muscle of the womb (uterus). They are not cancerous, but can give rise to symptoms such as heavy periods, and may then need surgical removal. Small fibroids which are not causing trouble are often left alone, subject to regular examination by doctor or gynaecologist.

Fibrositis. A painful condition of rheumatic type in muscle or related tissue. True disease of fibrous tissue, as implied by the name, is not very common, and the name is often applied to the combination of painful muscle spasm and adhesions in the lower back and shoulder girdle related to *spondylosis*. Pain of this type lasting a few days may follow a strain, excessive exercise, chilling, or influenza-like infections. Application of heat (see *Hot Water Bottles*) and a course of *aspirin* or *paracetamol* tablets may reasonalby be tried for a week. This will also allow time for the appearance of the rash of shingles (see *Herpes*) which sometimes mimics fibrositis. If trouble persists, a doctor should be consulted (C).

Finger, poisoned. Inflammation of the flesh of the finger by germs which have got below the skin, either through a small and perhaps invisible crack or scratch, or from penetration of a splinter or other foreign body.

First felt as a throbbing discomfort, it soon becomes a pain severe enough to prevent sleep. The part is swollen, red, and very tender, and if it is not treated promptly the bone of the fingertip may be damaged. The doctor should be consulted so that antibiotic treatment may be considered (S). Meanwhile:

1. No squeezing, pricking, or poking.
2. Rest the finger as much as possible.
3. *Hot bathing* every hour or two.

Paronychia, in which the inflammation is confined to the nail fold, takes a different form. The infecting germs may enter through torn cuticle or may complicate a settled infection of the nail fold, sometimes spread from athlete's foot or infection of the genital region. A simple primary infection will respond to hot bathing by forming a white or yellow blister containing pus round the nail fold. The doctor may be able to release the pus painlessly, and the inflammation then soon settles (S). If inflammation is being maintained by fungus or other transferred infection, the original sources of infection will have to be eradicated. Note here, that though hot bathing is a good short-term treatment for acute infection of the nail fold, it plays no part in the subsequent treatment of fungus infection, which requires the part to be kept completely dry during several weeks of treatment (S).

First Aid. Items of first aid are described under the following headings: *Abrasions, Burns, Bleeding, Cuts, Dressings, Drowning, Electric Shock, Eye, Fainting, Fracture, Gas, Injuries, Poisoning, Unconsciousness* and *Wounds;* it is generally agreed that the best way to learn first aid is to attend a course of practical instruction given by the local branch of the British Red Cross Society or St John Ambulance Brigade; in Scotland by St Andrew's Ambulance Association. These organizations publish their own instruction manuals.

Anyone needing to learn first aid without attending a course should read *New Essential First Aid* by Doctors A. Ward Gardner and P. J. Roylance (Pan Books), which is very clear and easily remembered.

First Aid

Suggested contents of a Household Medicine and First Aid Cup-board:

100 ml of 10 per cent solution of cetrimide in water. Note on label 'Dilute ten times with warm water before use.'

5 cm crepe bandage.

1 Triangular bandage (arm sling).

2 7.5 cm cotton conforming bandages, roller.

2 5 cm cotton conforming bandages, roller.

2 2.5 cm cotton bandages.

250 g cotton wool.

2 1-metre packets of sterilized gauze.

10 sterilized gauze swabs (7.5 cm square) individually wrapped.

Tin of 10 paraffin gauze squares. Take as required, using splinter forceps sterilized by boiling for five minutes.

Reel of 2.5 cm Elastoplast.

Reel of 1.25 cm zinc oxide plaster.

Packet of assorted adhesive dressing strips.

1 of each large, medium and small compressed wound dressings, BPC.

25 ml *Proflavine Cream*.

100 g *Bicarbonate of Soda*.

100 ml Calamine Lotion.

25 *Aspirin* or *paracetamol* tablets and 25 children's aspirin tablets. Foil-wrapped if possible, otherwise they will need renewal every few months.

200 ml *Kaolin Mixture* — renew every two or three months.

50 g *Magnesium Trisilicate* Compound Powder in airtight jar, or

25 *Magnesium Trisilicate* Compound Tablets BPC.

15 ml (i.e. one dose) of Ipecacuanha emetic draught, paediatric, BPC 1973 (quote this rigmarole in full when buying it, and see that it is so labelled). For use, see *Poisoning*.

6 Safety pins, assorted.

Dressing Scissors and Splinter Forceps, both to be boiled in water for five minutes before and after use.

Note-pad and pencil. 5 ml measuring spoon.

All kept under lock and key. Label all containers clearly, including doses and diluting instructions.

The cost of these items is not negligible, and quantities could be reduced for small households.

Fits (see *Convulsions, Epilepsy, Fainting*).

Flat Foot. To understand this it may help to remember that we have developed from ape-like animals who walked four-legged in trees. Both hands and feet were used for this, and they were held in a slightly clawed or arched state to be ready to grasp the branch, the tendency to grasp on contact being 'built in'. Though this made for rapid progress, it would be a disadvantage if the thing grasped proved to be damaging — a thorny branch, for instance — and to reduce damage, the hands and feet were provided with means whereby, if pain was registered by palm or sole, the grasping muscles immediately relaxed to allow the limb to be withdrawn. This 'reflex' accounts for the immediate release of a plate which has been picked up and which proves to be unexpectedly hot. It is dropped so quickly that one is aware of it falling before knowing one has been burned. In the same way, a corn or verruca, an ill-fitting shoe or one with a nail in it, causing a footstep to be painful, leads to the relaxation of the muscles holding the arched toes in the grasping position. When the weight falls on the foot, the toes and small joints flatten out on the ground like the tracks of a tank, instead of providing a forward spring from the great toe for the next step. A shorter pace results, the flattened foot being carried forward in one piece and plonked down, still flat.

If this process continues, the muscles responsible for clawing the toes into arches lose their power and the three sprung arches connecting the heel, big toe, and little toe are lost. This is most obvious on the inner side of the foot, where most of the weight is taken on the highest arch, and its collapse causes the ankle joint to bend out of the straight, a position which affects the muscular balance of the whole leg. Flatness of the short cross arch between the first and fifth toes can produce metatarsalgia, pain due to pressure on the nerves serving the toes. Temporary flat foot often follows resumption of walking after an illness, due to weakness of the leg muscles.

Some children pass through a few years during which the leg muscles are relatively weak, allowing the inner arch to fall and the ankle joint to bend. A knock knee develops as a correction to this, and there is uncertainty at present whether this corrects itself naturally, or whether corrective treatment is needed.

All forms of flat foot call for medical advice (C). If the wearing of wedged shoes is advised, it is important that they should be worn from getting up until going to bed. There is a temptation to leave off the shoes — which should be lace-up ones — in summer or to use wedged sandals instead. In the writer's experience, the time thus lost has to be paid for later.

Treatment of flat foot aims at correcting the original cause, by removing verrucas, etc, and ensuring good fit of footwear; then strengthening the supporting muscles of the arches by exercises and electrical treatment. The exercises are simple, but success depends on carrying them out as instructed as a daily routine over a long period.

Anyone with a tendency to flat foot should avoid the extremes of fashion in footwear (unless a broad toe and straight inner edge happen to be in fashion!) and should aim to have roomy comfortable working shoes for daily wear, reserving the smarter ones for special appearances.

Flatulence (see *Wind*).

'Flooding'. Usually used to describe excessive loss at the time of the monthly period, or a sudden massive vaginal loss at any time. See the entry 'Bleeding from Vagina' at the end of *Bleeding, internal*.

Flushing or **Blushing.** Flushing with anger or embarrassment may in the past have had some biological value in warning an enemy that he had gone too far, and so giving him the chance to climb down without undergoing the hazard of a fight. It is now only a social nuisance and steps should be taken to avoid the situations which cause it. On reflection, it will often be found that blushing follows the disclosure of oneself in a slightly adverse light, and it will usually be possible further to discern the minor tactical error which allows one to be found in such a position, and to avoid it. The entries *Anxiety*, *Contemplation*, and *Relaxation* will help.

A permanently flushed condition of the face may be due to illness, and the doctor should be consulted (C). The commonest cause, acne rosacea, can usually be controlled if the treatment is followed conscientiously. Many women experience flushing at or around the *menopause*. It can often be helped by simple treatment (C).

Food Poisoning. The result of eating food infected by *germs*. Usually takes the form of acute *gastritis* or *gastroenteritis*, and is treated in the same way. The germs causing salmonella poisoning inhabit the excreta of rats, mice, birds, and human *carriers*, and contamination occurs through faults in storage, merchandizing, or service. As thorough cooking destroys the infection, trouble more often arises from cold cooked meats, etc, which have been allowed to cool gradually, allowing a period of raised temperature during which any bacteria not killed in the cooking can multiply and colonize the meat. The disease is commonest in the third quarter of the year, when contamination by flies is most likely, and in this it differs from the virus gastroenteritis of the winter months. The latter tends to affect members of a family at intervals of several days, as each catches it from the other in turn, whereas salmonella usually strikes everybody susceptible 12 to 24 hours after the food has been eaten. When symptoms start within a few hours, staphylococcal poisoning is the likely cause. Here, staphylococcal bacteria from a boil or septic sore on a handler infect the food, producing a poison which causes the gastroenteritis. Although the staphylococci are killed by thorough cooking, the poison they have already produced is not destroyed, and the severity of the poisoning thus depends on how long the staphylococci have been at work between reaching the food and being cooked.

Some rare forms of food poisoning such as botulism give

rise to illness so severe that the urgent need for medical care is obvious (U).

Prevention 1 The thorough washing of hands with soap and hot water after using the lavatory and before starting any culinary operation.
2 Testing of all food handlers to exclude carriers of disease.
3 Scrupulous cleansing of utensils.
4 Control of flies.

Foreskin. A retractable sleeve of skin which protects the end of the penis. At birth, the foreskin may not be completely separated from the underlying penis, becoming so gradually during the first months or years of life. As a routine, a baby's foreskin should be pulled back as far as it will go without forcing, every time he is bathed. If this is persevered in, the skin will be gradually stretched as it separates, and it will finally be possible to retract it easily behind the ridge of the tip of the penis, cleanse, and then pull it forward again. This should be done as part of the bathing routine, after most other parts have been washed, but not at the very end, to avoid drawing particular attention to the organ; probably best done just before cleansing between the buttocks, which should end the bath. Try to make the process just another item in the routine, not making a perceptible effort or 'nerving' oneself to do it — it is much better not to persist for that day if the attempt at retraction fails the first time. There is no great hurry, *unless* at any time the retracted foreskin gets stuck behind the ridge of the penis and cannot be brought forward. Should this happen, keep calm. Grasp the roll of foreskin between first and second figners, as if holding the neck of a bottle before pushing the cork in with the thumb. Now do just that — push the tip of the penis gently backwards with the thumb into the ring of foreskin. Maintain the gentle pressure for a minute or two, when the collapsible tip will reduce in size and slip back through the roll of foreskin, which will then be drawn gently forwards. In an adult, the fingers and thumbs of both hands will be needed, the thumbs gently compressing the tip from both sides. Should this manoeuvre fail, the case must be brought to medical care in the course of a few hours, otherwise damage may occur (S or D).

Occasionally, at birth, the foreskin is so tight that it obstructs the passage of urine. This is rare, but it is easily dealt with by the doctor. The foreskin can become the seat of infection, trapped between foreskin and penis. This rarely happens if ordinary cleansing is practised. When it does, medical treatment is needed (S). (See also *Circumcision*.)

Fracture. The breaking or cracking of a bone. A *Compound (or Open) Fracture* occurs when the broken bone, or the object causing it, penetrates the skin, opening a channel for infection of the bone. In *Simple (Closed) Fracture* the broken bone is not exposed to the air. It can be serious in other ways, as by causing internal bleeding or damaging an organ.

The first treatment of fracture is that of the general injury situation which may have produced it, and is covered under *Injuries* and *Shock*.

Freckles. Small areas which pigment more rapidly on exposure to sunlight than the surrounding skin. They are thus more prominent in summer than winter. Fortunately, many people find them attractive; and as there is at present no way of removing them, their possessors should cultivate an attitude of mind based on this. They can, of course, be concealed or disguised by make-up for formal appearances, particularly in artificial light, if it is thought necessary.

Frostbite. The severest form of cold injury, of which *Chilblains* are one of the mildest, results in cutting off the blood supply of the affected part, so that it turns white. The treatment is to immerse the part in hot water at 110–115 degrees F (43–46 degrees C) for 20 to 40 minutes, until the normal colour returns. This temperature is about as hot as can be tolerated when tested with normal (unbitten) skin. Both before and after treatment, the part must be handled very gently, as its circulation has been damaged, and the older treatments of massage, rubbing with snow, etc, are no longer advised. If hot water treatment cannot be given on the spot, it is better to get the patient to where it can, rather than waste time on other measures. (But see under *Exposure* — a decision based on priorities may have to be taken.)

Fungus. A large group of vegetable organisms widespread throughout nature. The visible group includes *toadstools* and *mushrooms*. The invisible ones can infect the skin of men and animals, giving rise to *ringworm, athlete's foot*, etc. (See *Ringworm*).

Gas or Fume Poisoning. The gas responsible for most fume poisoning is carbon monoxide. This is contained in coal and coke fumes, and motor engine exhausts, but not in 'natural' or 'North Sea' gas, so that the latter does not poison as coal gas used to, though it can explode violently, and if there is enough of it to displace the air from a confined space, it will suffocate.

A person unconscious in a fume-filled room is assumed to be suffering from carbon monoxide poisoning. As soon as the situation is recognized, withdraw from the room at once and shut the door. If any other responsible person is present, ask him to call an ambulance or doctor, stating the case as one of carbon monoxide poisoning. Make sure he knows the correct address. Now prepare for a twenty second reconnaissance of the room. Take three long slow breaths, holding in the third, and open the door. If an engine is running, turn it off. After ten seconds, start to breath out slowly through pursed lips, making it last another ten seconds, by which time you are leaving the room and closing the door. You should have had time to get to a window and open it, or inspect its fastenings. At worst you should know if the window can be opened or must be broken, and this should occupy the next twenty seconds sortie. Do remember your responsibility to people who may be injured by falling glass, and act accordingly. If the window *must* be broken, one or two panes at top *and* bottom will give the quickest ventilation of the room.

Get back your breath, repeat the 3 breaths, go in and pull the patient out by the heels, using every care possible to avoid injury. Close the door. If the patient is not breathing, *artificial respiration* is started immediately (together with cardiac massage as described under *Drowning*, if indicated), having first made sure the patient's mouth and airway are not obstructed by dislodged teeth, vomit, carpet fluff, etc. If the window fastening is easy, there may be a chance to call from the open window for help before removing the patient. Do not spend long over it, for every minute counts in starting artificial respiration.

With artificial respiration under way, the course of events depends on the circumstances:

1. If a message has been sent for an ambulance, continue artificial respiration until ambulance crew take over.
2. If in a situation where no ambulance or doctor is available, continue artificial respiration, employing relays of helpers if any are available, until patient recovers or is obviously dead (see *Death*).
3. If dealing with the emergency alone, artificial respiration should be continued at least half an hour before breaking off to call for any help which may be within one or two minutes summons. If none such is available, continue as for (2).

With the patient breathing satisfactorily, with or without the need for artificial respiration, he should be sent directly to hospital or be seen on the spot by a doctor.

Gastric Ulcer (see also *Peptic Ulcer*). The destruction of a small area of the inner lining of the stomach. A patient who has abdominal pain at a definite interval after taking food, for several days or a few weeks at a time, with intervals of freedom from pain lasting several weeks or even months, may have a gastric ulcer, or some other complaint. He should take medical advice (**C**).

A patient who has, or has had, a gastric ulcer should never take *aspirin*, as it can aggravate the ulcer.

There are two occasional complications of gastric ulcer when medical help is urgent:

1. **Vomiting blood.** (See *Bleeding, internal* — U or UU, depending on severity.)

124 Gastritis (Inflammation of Stomach)

2 Leakage through the wall of the stomach where the ulcer has weakened it, allowing the acid gastric juice to escape. This causes very severe pain in the abdomen and is a surgical emergency. The patient must be brought under medical care in the course of the next hour or two (UU), and if the doctor cannot reach him he must be got within that time to the nearest hospital that has surgical facilities.

No food or drink to be given in either of these situations while awaiting medical help.

Gastritis (Inflammation of Stomach) can be *acute*, lasting a few hours or days or *chronic*, lasting weeks or months.

Acute: A feeling of nausea and fullness in the upper abdomen followed by vomiting, often repeated. The attack may last for several hours, so that the stomach is emptied and bitter yellow or green fluid (bile) is vomited. Sometimes, the attack is followed after some hours by left-sided lower abdominal pains and diarrhoea, or these may start soon after the vomiting. Vomiting that starts after several days of constipation may be caused by a hold-up in the bowel, and if it persists more than a few hours, getting worse rather than better, or if brown, foul smelling matter is vomited, the doctor should be called (U or D). For treatment of acute gastritis, see *Gastroenteritis*.

Occasional confusion arises when nausea and vomiting accompany pain felt behind the breast bone in the middle of the chest, at the start of a *coronary attack*. Generally in such cases it is the pain which the patient complains of, the vomiting being the lesser of his troubles. This pain may be felt in the central upper abdomen just below the end of the breast bone, or may extend upwards from the centre of the chest to one or both shoulders or arms, and the patient may be pale, or grey, with cold hands. If heart trouble is suspected, the patient should be rested in bed, propped up if necessary, and the doctor sent for (U or UU).

Chronic gastritis is a diagnosis made by the doctor after examination and such tests as he judges necessary. It is not a subject for home treatment.

Gastroenteritis. One of the few abdominal pains which it is usually safe for the amateur to diagnose is the colic accompanying an acute attack of diarrhoea. This is felt low in the belly and to the left side, and feels like a painful exaggeration of the normal urge to open the bowels. The spasms last from a few seconds to a few minutes and may be very severe, leading to sweating and occasionally fainting. Between spasms there is no pain. Such attacks often form part of an attack of gastroenteritis when, following a feeling of nausea, the patient vomits several times. Sometimes the vomiting and diarrhoea coincide.

Treatment Realize that in this situation the patient has a sore throat the size of a 2-lb. bag (his stomach) leading to one several yards long (the intestine). Both organs have a keen interest in ridding themselves of their contents, and the stomach will react by vomiting anything swallowed, or by passing it into the intestine, where it will start a spasm of movement leading to emptying of the bowel. Try a mixture of equal parts of cold milk and water, taking one sip at a time and warming it in the mouth before swallowing. If *magnesium trisilicate* powder is available, take half a level 5 ml spoonful (or 2 crushed magnesium trisilicate tablets) with a little of the milk/water, repeating in 2 hours' time. Failing these, half a 5 ml spoonful of bicarbonate of soda can be taken during the first half hour, but not later, and should not be repeated. If vomiting persists, one or two 5 ml spoonfuls of brandy, whisky, or gin, diluted if desired but better not, slowly swallowed and repeated after half an hour. This last measure is also helpful in diarrhoea and colic in the absence of vomiting, when it should be combined with the taking of two 5 ml spoonfuls of *kaolin mixture* every three hours to a total of four doses. (All these are adult doses.)

A guarded *hot water bottle* against the soles of the feet and another to the lower abdomen will help. Old hands in the tropics advised lying for ten minutes in a hot bath with the water covering the abdomen.

Once the attack has passed, normal feeing should be resumed after 24 hours of light intake. For this, the milk mixture is increased in strength and size. Once whole milk can be retained, thin bread and butter, jelly, blancmange, mashed banana with milk, cereal, *all cold* and in *small helpings*, taken every 1 or 2 hours.

For lingering diarrhoea, grated dessert apple allowed to brown on a plate and then eaten a few spoonfuls at a time, is helpful, but see under *Diarrhoea* for cases which continue more than a few days.

The bowels may not act for 2 or 3 days after an attack of diarrhoea, but will normally start again of their own accord without help.

Continued alternating diarrhoea and constipation can be caused by disease of the rectum and demand medical consultation (C).

Before going abroad, ask your doctor for a prescription for suitable treatment for an attack. You will have to pay for it, as it is not available under the National Health Service.

German Measles (Rubella). One of the infectious diseases, usually mild. Its importance lies in the risk of harm to the developing baby if a pregnant mother catches it during the first four months of her pregnancy It is best to have medical advice in all cases in which the mother has been in contact with the disease during the first four months of pregnancy (S), as the situation is complicated by the tendency of several different virus infections to produce a rash resembling German measles, and a serum test may be needed.

In the typical case, after three days off colour, the patient develops a finely blotched rash spreading from the back of the neck over the whole body. There may be signs of a mild cold, but the persistent cough of true measles is absent, and the rash is lighter in colour. At the very back of the skull, towards the neck, several lumps like lentils or small peas may be felt under the skin.

Unless there is need to confirm the diagnosis in girls or early pregnancy, the average case hardly merits a visit from the doctor, the patient being rested until the rash fades, then kept away from other people for a further week.

Vaccination against rubella is now advised for all girls in their early teens, and for unvaccinated women of child bearing age, whether or not they are believed to have had the disease.

Incubation Period: 14–21 days.

Quarantine: 23 days, but child contacts are not nowadays excluded from school.

Germs. A useful term for the description of microscopically small organisms which cause disease. As usually encountered, these are:

1. Bacteria, minute single-celled plants such as streptococci (causing eg, tonsillitis), straphylococci (boils), and bacilli (cystitis), which can be seen with the highest magnification of an ordinary microscope. Mostly, they can be grown easily in incubators and studied with ordinary laboratory apparatus. Most can be killed by antibiotics.
2. Viruses, very much smaller, invisible by ordinary methods and unrecognizable except after lengthy investigation in special laboratories. Not only do they invade the body as bacteria do, but they enter into its cells and convert the chemical processes of the body to their own purposes. For the most part they are unaffected by antibiotics and have to be overcome by the body's natural resistance. Viruses cause such illnesses as common cold, measles, and poliomyelitis.

Giddiness. The most severe form, in which the patient feels that he or his surroundings are rotating or tilting, is described under *Vertigo*. A feeling of muzziness or confusion lasting a few seconds usually results from a reduction of the blood supply to the brain. In some people this is constitutional, due to delay in the automatic shut-down of circulation in the lower part of the body when rising from the sitting or lying position. This short delay allows the circulating blood to fall back from the brain until it is pushed up again by a few forceful beats of the heart. Anyone who is conscious of this tendency can prevent trouble by taking a little longer in rising from the lying position, and by clenching the muscles of the calves, thighs, and buttocks as they stand up. (This trick is also useful in dealing with a threat of faintness which sometimes occurs after standing still for some time.)

Of course, if the pumping action of the heart is weakened, a similar temporary loss of brain circulation will be produced on standing, and one should take medical advice if the tendency to giddiness starts in someone not previously subject to it.

A frequent cause of giddiness or even fainting in older people is the kinking of two arteries which carry blood up the back of the neck to the brain. This happens in a rheumatic neck, when throwing the head back to look up, while hanging out clothes, opening a high window, or reading a newspaper through bifocal glasses. A knowledge of the cause allows one to avoid the effect.

Gland. An organ which produces and releases fluid into or out of the system. Thus the glands of the stomach lining secrete digestive juices into the stomach, sweat glands of the skin excrete sweat when the skin needs to cool, sebaceous glands make oil in hair roots; while the pituitary, thyroid, and others inject variable amounts of very potent internal secretions ('hormones') into the circulation, which regulate the action of the heart, liver, sugar supply, etc, according to the varying needs of the body.

What are often called lymph glands, soft, bean-shaped objects under the skin of the neck, armpit, and groin — hardly meet this description, and are now more often called lymph nodes. They act as check-points on the drainage system of the throat, limbs, etc, stopping the passage of any germs which may be trying to penetrate the body's defences after getting through the tonsils, or a cut in the skin. The lymph nodes under the angle of the jaw are often swollen and tender in the course of a throat infection, and this may spread to the other nodes in the neck; the condition often called 'glands in the neck'. They usually subside within a week or two of the throat infection. If they do not, the doctor should be consulted. A painful lymph node in armpit or groin, the presence of a cut, boil, or *whitlow*, and a faint pink line wandering up the corresponding limb is a signal for medical treatment the same day (S or D). Meanwhile, *hot bathing* to the node and to the original site of infection, every hour or two. Enlarged lymph nodes found anywhere in the body should be regarded as *lumps* and taken to the doctor (S). (See also *Stye* and *Pain, armpit*.)

Glandular Fever. An infection of lymph nodes (see above) by a group of viruses. May be suspected if a feverish sore throat with 'glands' in the neck becomes progressively worse in the course of a week or so, or returns a few days after having cleared up. Swollen lymph nodes may be felt in groin or armpit and the patient may become jaundiced (D or V, according to severity).

Glaucoma. An eye disorder of middle and later life in which an increase of pressure inside the eye damages the sight — permanently, unless treatment is prompt. The acute type with sudden onset of severe aching pain in and around an inflamed eye, sometimes leading to vomiting and prostration, obviously needs medical help (S or D), but the gradual onset of chronic glaucoma is more difficult to recognize. A slow deterioration of sight, occasional neuralgia over one eye, and the appearance of a 'halo' or of rings of light seen around lamps when walking at night, are all warning signs (C). (See also *Sight* and *Screening Tests*.)

Goitre. Swelling of the thyroid gland at the front of the neck. Needs medical advice (S).

Gonorrhoea. A very common *veneral disease*. Within ten days (usually, sometimes longer) of intercourse, the victim feels a scalding pain on passing water, varying from mild to very intense. In a few days a discharge of pus may be seen from the inflamed urinary passage. Before this the patient should be in the hands of his or her doctor or have attended a *VD centre* for the earlier treatment is started the better the chance of complete cure, and of avoiding the serious complications that arise in untreated gonorrhoea. Strict cooperation in treatment is essential, as is attendance for the checks periodically advised, particularly the serum test at six months for possible *syphilis*, as a partner who had unsuspected gonorrhoea may also have had this more serious disease.

Medical advice should be taken before resuming intercourse, to avoid further spread of infection.

Signs of infection in the female can be slight, and may not be noticed.

Anyone whose partner develops gonorrhoea within a month of intercourse should seek a full examination.

Gout. An inherited constitutional defect leading to the presence of too much uric acid in the body. This finds its way into joints, particularly the great toe joints, and renders them liable to attacks of gout.

In a typical attack, the patient is awakened in the night with severe pain in the toe, which soon becomes hot, shiny, swollen, and very tender to touch. The attack abates under treatment in the course of some days. For first aid treatment, *aspirin* or *paracetamol* tablets should be taken in full doses, as shown under their separate headings, and a cradle should be improvised to keep the bedclothes off the feet. Cooling lotion such as calamine or Eau-de-Cologne with water half and half can be applied to the painful part. In the morning the doctor is notified (D).

Many gouty people can keep themselves free from trouble by avoiding the foods which produce most uric acid in the body, such as liver, sweetbreads, kidney, meat extracts, fish roes, and by avoiding over-indulgence in meaty foods. The effect of alcohol varies, but attacks are sometimes brought on by a rich meal with alcoholic drinks. Routine preventive treatment with tablets may be advised, and is effective if followed conscientiously. Some gouty attacks occur towards the end of a feverish illness, such as influenza, and there may be two factors at work — the fever releases uric acid in the system, and the continued catching of the toes in the bedclothes irritates the joints. It is possible that the last may

- **If a patient is not within the scope of home care, or worsens in spite of it, or if there is any uncertainty, a doctor should be consulted.**

account for attacks at other times, for these joints often have a restricted range of movement, and if the toe is forced beyond that when the patient turns over in bed, the forcible manipulation of the joint could cause inflammation. It is a useful precaution to make the foot of the bed loosely and to include a bolster in it to allow free rotation of the feet.

Growing Pains (see under *Rheumatic Fever*).

Gums. Inflammation, with pain, redness, and ulceration, sometimes spreading to the tongue and lips, and offensive breath, is usually gingivitis, attributable to faulty dental hygiene, or lowered resistance from a variety of causes. Expert opinion now doubts if it is caught from infected utensils as was formerly believed.

A dentist should be consulted as soon as possible. Meanwhile, thorough mouth washing with one part of '20 volume' hydrogen peroxide to three of warm water, every four hours, and the use of soft tooth picks night and morning. The patient's toilet gear, crockery, and eating utensils must be kept separate and either destroyed or sterilized by boiling for 20 minutes once he is clear of infection.

The victim may persuade himself that he has scurvy and waste time and money taking vitamin C, but scurvy is very rare in this country. Sore gums in anyone working with lead or lead compounds should be seen by the patient's or the works' doctor (S).

One or more small painful ulcers, on tongue, gums, or mouth in an otherwise healthy mouth are aphthous ulcers. They usually clear up in the course of ten days; if not, show them to your doctor for confirmation of the diagnosis. Both cause and cure are unknown, and some people are prone to repeated attacks. Rubbing each ulcer gently with a paste made from an aspirin tablet and a drop of water, two or three times a day, brings relief.

Pyorrhoea is a progressive infection of the edges of the gums, which have a grey, rotten look and seem not to fit closely round the teeth. Dental treatment is essential.

Haemorrhage (see Bleeding).

Haemorrhoids (Piles). One of the penalties paid by man for walking on two legs instead of four. The weight of the abdominal organs causes pressure on the veins running up under the lining of the rectum, so that they become engorged and bulge into the cavity of the bowel, where they can be carried down by a passing motion and trapped outside. The blood in them clots, and the very tender swellings protrude from the anus. In the acute stage it may be necessary to rest several days while the congestion disperses and the pile shrivels. Before this stage is reached, the pile may come down temporarily and withdraw of its own accord; or may be persuaded to do so by gentle pressure with a pad of cotton wool wrung out of hot water. At other times, the only sign of haemorrhoids may be the passage of blood when the bowel acts.

Haemorrhoids are a matter for medical advice, so that more serious trouble can be excluded (C, or V in an acute attack). A *hot pack* to the tender part, repeated every hour or two and *aspirin* or *paracetamol* tablets will relieve pain as first aid in an acute attack. It is believed that a high residue diet (bran and vegetable roughage) reduces the tendency to piles.

Halitosis (Foul Breath). Can arise anywhere between the lips and the lungs. It does not often arise from digestive causes.

1. Infectious ulcers of the lips, mouth, and gums. (See *Gingivitis*, see page 131.)
2. Decaying food trapped between the teeth, particularly the front teeth, may not be removed by brushing, and the spaces should be cleared with dental picks, bought from the chemist, before the teeth are brushed. At first this will be necessary after each meal, but can usually be restricted to night and morning when the situation has been brought under control.
3. Decayed and broken-down teeth. Until these have been dentally cleared, foul breath must be expected. Inadequate cleansing of dentures is another cause.
4. Chronically enlarged and infected tonsils. These can be

treated temporarily with swabs of cotton wool on sticks, moistened with 'Listerine', twice a day, but removal of tonsils is the only permanent cure.
5 When arising from *sinus* or antrum infection, will clear when the cause is dealt with (C).
6 A very unpleasant breath is found in some patients suffering from a chronic infection of the bronchial tubes called bronchiectasis. In severe cases it can be almost unbearable for the bystanders. In so far as treatment is possible, it is that of the bronchiectasis (C).

Hallucinations. Symptoms of mental illness. The patient believes he is hearing, seeing, smelling, feeling, etc, things which do not happen or exist. The increasingly successful treatment of mental illness makes it important to bring such patients under medical care as soon as possible, both for treatment and to prevent the risk of suicide or violence which sometimes exists. Those close to the patient have a real problem in deciding how to deal with his account of his experiences, whether by accepting them without comment or demurring. In general, it is best to adopt that line of approach which is judged least likely further to disturb the patient. If he can be persuaded to visit his doctor, the latter should be informed previously of the abnormalities observed, as the patient may give out that he is consulting the doctor on some unconnected matter. If the situation is obviously degenerating quickly, the doctor should be asked to call (D, U, or UU) and the message should give him some idea of the situation, as it may be inadvisable for him to seem to be discussing the patient with others on his arrival.

Hallux Valgus. A condition in which the great toe is angled towards the outside of the foot, producing a prominence of the great toe joint on which a *bunion* may form. The cause is debatable and it seems that some people may be born with a tendency to hallux valgus, the onset of which may be delayed or prevented by:

1 Keeping children in broad-toed straight inner sided shoes until social pressures make it impracticable.

2. Early correction of tendency to flat foot and/or knock knee by such measures as the doctor advises.
3. Teach children to walk with feet pointing forwards, not toeing out. Every effort should be made to persuade an adolescent threatened with hallux valgus to avoid the extremes of shoe fashion.

Once established, treatment is by orthopaedic surgery (C).

Handicap (see *Disability*).

Hay Fever. A manifestation of allergy in which the subject is sensitive to the pollen of grass or flowers. It produces swelling of the lining of the nose and irritation of the membranes lining the eyelids, leading to nasal obstruction, sneezing, and itching eyes. The intensity varies with the amount of pollen in the air and hay fever is, of course, seasonal, only occurring when the causative plant is pollinating.

Similar sensitivities to house dust, cat fur, etc, can operate all the year round, producing 'allergic rhinitis', of which seasonal hay fever is one example.

Apart from steps to avoid areas of high pollen concentration, treatment is medical, by means of antihistamine preparations, insufflations, or by a course of immunizing injections the previous winter. Although these courses have been reduced in length, they still last several weeks, and it is best to get in touch with the doctor in the autumn so that the necessary tests at an allergy clinic can be arranged in time to allow completion of the course. Only in exceptional circumstances should a child or young person be made to undertake such a course unless they volunteer for it themselves having fully understood what is involved.

Headache (see *Pain in head*).

Heartburn. As usually understood, discomfort felt behind the lower part of the breast bone after taking food. Although it happens occasionally to most people after injudicious feeding, when half a teaspoonful of bicarbonate of soda in a little water will often relieve it, some are particularly prone to it, so that it forms a continuing complaint. Then, it is usually due to acid gastric juice being forced upwards into the gullet, and is more likely to happen if the gap in the diaphragm muscle through which the gullet passes is too large, so that the upper part of the stomach is squeezed by the diaphragm. This will happen on bending down, as in gardening or sweeping, and is worse if there is much abdominal fat. The diagnosis is made by X-ray examination which may reveal the so-called 'hiatus hernia' in the diaphragm.

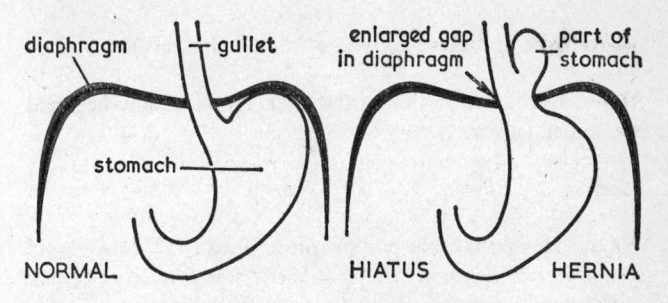

Diagram: NORMAL (diaphragm, gullet, stomach) vs. HIATUS HERNIA (enlarged gap in diaphragm, part of stomach)

Most cases are minor or trivial in effect and may give no trouble if excess weight is shed (by reducing the intake of bread, potatoes, sugar, sweets, cakes, pastries, and other carbohydrate foods) and if frequent small feeds are taken in place of a few main meals. If these measures do not help, consult your doctor (**C**).

It is useless, and may be harmful, to treat an established case of 'heartburn' by taking bicarbonate of soda or other similar remedies without professional advice.

Heart Disease. (For an illustration of the heart, see page 85.)

Many more people fear that they have heart disease than have it. As the heart is an essential organ, and partly because of its ancient and spurious reputation as the seat of emotion, it is natural that anyone prone to excessive anxiety should fear and believe that the heart is diseased. The presence of true heart disease or weakness is seldom suspected by the sufferer, but is found by the doctor on examination.

If you fear that you may have heart disease, don't hang about worrying; go to your doctor, (C) and tell him (1) what you feel wrong and (2) what you fear is wrong. He will question you about the first and examine you. As a result he may be able to reassure you as to the second, or he may ask for further investigations. If these are negative, you will be reassured and your fears should disappear. If they do not, the chances are very strong that your complaint is not heart disease but over-anxiety, and this in turn may need medical treatment. (See also *Palpitation* and *Anxiety*.)

Heatstroke and **Heat Exhaustion** (see *Sunstroke*).

Hepatitis. Inflammation of the liver. For infectious hepatitis see under *Jaundice*.

Hernia (see *Rupture, Vomiting, Heartburn*).

Herpes zoster and **Herpes simplex.** Two conditions caused when nerves supplying the skin are irritated by a virus.

Herpes zoster (Shingles) is caused by the same virus as chickenpox. It causes a trail of small blisters in a zone one or two inches wide which usually runs horizontally half round the trunk (if head or limb is affected, the pattern is different). Pain is often felt in the affected part for several days before the rash appears. The blisters dry and heal in the course of two or three weeks; second attacks are unusual. Virus is contained in the blisters, so contaminated dressings should be burned, and old cotton vests worn, so that they can be burned after the attack.

Early treatment of the rash is with calamine lotion, dabbed on every four hours or so. It is important to control the pain as far as possible by taking *aspirin* or *paracetamol*, in the doses mentioned under their headings, as this helps to prevent the tiresome neuralgia which can otherwise last for months after an attack. Once the scabs have dropped from the scars, these should be lightly massaged with the finger tips and a little olive oil, or preferably be given vibro-massage with the rubber studded pad of an electric massager for five to ten minutes two or three times daily, to combat the development of neuralgia. The doctor should be consulted early in all but the mildest cases (S or V).

Herpes simplex is usually seen as a 'cold sore' on the face and differs from shingles in being less severe and in its tendency to return in the same place for several years. Dabbing with calamine lotion or surgical spirit is usually all that is needed.

Both kinds of herpes can affect the eyes, and any pain or inflammation occurring in the course of an attack should have medical attention (S).

Caution 1 It is unwise and can be hazardous, to treat either type of herpes with lotions or ointments left over from treatment of some other complaint. In the eyes particularly, a dangerous flare-up of the disease has occurred after doing so.

2 Do not expose the skin to direct sunlight if a cold sore is present, as the combination of sunburn and herpes simplex can produce a troublesome sensitivity rash.

Hiatus Hernia (see *Heartburn*).

Hiccup. A spasmodic contraction of the diaphragm muscle repeated at intervals. In the index of most textbooks of medicine, it is only mentioned as a complication of certain acute illnesses, which would seem to suggest that the ordinary uncomplicated hiccup seldom comes to medical notice. The cause is not known; some are more prone to it than others, and some attacks seem to be related to distension of the stomach by a heavy meal. Many people will adopt one or other of the popular ploys, such as breathing into and out of a paper bag, or drinking water in various unusual positions. If such fail, lie back in an easy chair with the head supported and the feet on a stool to flex the thighs. Concentrate on relaxing the spine and abdominal muscles so that the belly moves easily with each breath. Turn on the radio or gramophone fairly loudly, or read a book, for a quarter of an hour.

Very rarely, hiccup continuing for several hours, particularly in an older person, can cause exhaustion and needs medical treatment (D).

Honeymoon. A happy honeymoon can be expected if both partners have done their homework — preferably from the same book* — and when both have agreed in advance whether to practise contraception; and if so, how.

Two or three months before marriage is not too soon to take advice about this (see *Contraception*), particularly if oral contraception ('The Pill') is under consideration.
(*See *Marriage*).

Hot bathing and **Hot packs.** Both treat and relieve acute inflammation; that is, a hot, painful, swollen, often reddened condition of a part (such as a finger-tip) or area of skin (early boil, septic mosquito bite, following a prick, etc).

Plain hot water or hot *isotonic saline* is used, and as hot as can comfortably be borne. For a finger, or other part that can be immersed, a deep bowl is filled with the hot fluid and after preliminary testing for temperature, the finger is immersed to cover the inflamed area. At first, it may have to be removed after a few seconds if the fluid is very hot, but gradually it can be kept in for longer at a time. As the fluid cools, it is reheated or renewed. The whole exercise should last about ten minutes and be repeated every two to four hours.

If the inflamed area can't be immersed, it is treated by wringing a square of towelling or such-like out of the hot water to free it of drips, testing it for safe heat on the back of the hand, then holding it against the inflamed area as long as the heat lasts, before repeating the process, for a total of ten minutes at a time, every two to four hours.

Hot Fomentations are not used nowadays, their place having been largely taken by *kaolin poultice*.

It is important to guard against scalding by preliminary testing as described above.

Hot Water Bottles. The use of these comfortable things needs more care than is sometimes realized. They should never be used for unconscious patients, nor in contact with a part which has lost its sense of touch or heat, or which the patient cannot move. When a patient is generally poorly, as with gastroenteritis or a 'chill', it is comforting to have a 'guarded' hot water bottle against the soles of the feet and/or the abdomen. A hot water bottle is 'guarded' in three ways:

1. When filled, the naked bottle is not too hot for the back of one's hand to bear.
2. It is then wrapped in its cover, or a towel, or blanket.
3. A metal stopper must be covered to prevent it touching the patient.

A hot water bottle which is to be used on the abdomen should not be more than half full, otherwise the weight of it will be uncomfortable.

A guarded hot water bottle is a good bedfellow to lumbago, stiff neck, and fibrositis, and is worth a trial in various rheumatic conditions. The use of much hotter water bottles for 'drawing' septic conditions should be only on medical advice.

Housemaid's Knee (Bursitis). Inflammation of the cushion of soft tissue in front of the knee, just below the kneecap. It happens when a part of the day's work is spent kneeling, with the weight forwards, as in scrubbing or polishing, so that it is concentrated on the knees rather than the shin. The vibration transmitted from the working arms plays a part. The skin is red, swollen, and tender, but the knee joint itself is not involved. If kneeling work is persisted in, the inflammation will not settle, and it may recur if such work is started too soon after an attack, or with insufficient cushioning.

Treatment consists in resting the legs for some days, applying *kaolin poultices* two or three times a day. Fluid or even pus may form and make its way to the surface along the core of the corn which sometimes forms on the skin of kneeling workers. Anything more than a mild attack needs medical advice (C or V).

Prevention A thick foam rubber kneeling pad should be made which allows the weight to be mainly taken below the knees, which project just beyond its edge. It should be cased in canvas to preserve its shape. The kneeling position should be changed

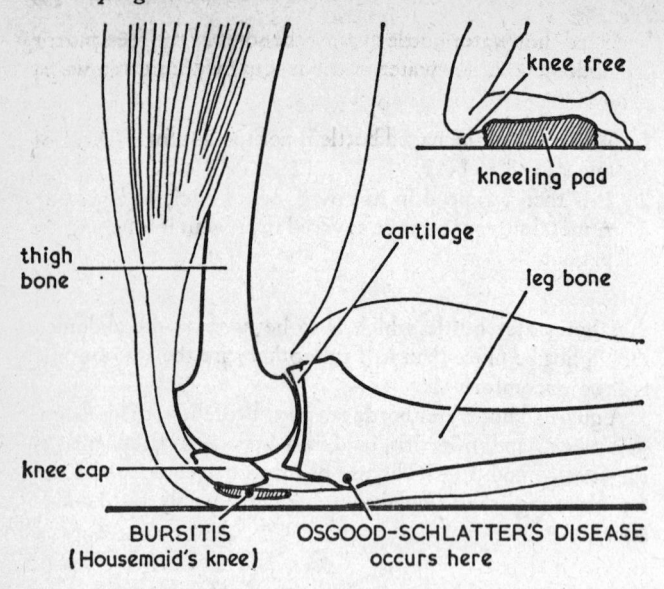

Labels on figure: knee free, kneeling pad, cartilage, leg bone, thigh bone, knee cap, BURSITIS (Housemaid's knee), OSGOOD-SCHLATTER'S DISEASE occurs here

The knee seen from the side

frequently to avoid over-stretching from one position. (See illustration, above.)

Hydrogen Peroxide. Usually bought in '20 volume' strength. **Note that it bleaches most colours.** It is a useful mouthwash for gingivitis, diluted one part with three of warm water, and in the same dilution will often stop a nose bleed, if a swab of cotton wool or ribbon gauze is soaked in it and pushed well up the nostril — always leave part of the swab sticking out, for easy removal. See *Gums*.

Hygiene, personal. Based on the principle that what the body gets rid of is best out of the way. Secretions and excretions retained on the skin soon become offensive, if they are not already so, and where skin surfaces are in contact (armpits, buttocks, and thighs) bacteria spread and multiply.

The following suggestions are for those doing moderate or light work in a temperate climate and are the minimum compatible with the comfort of others:

Scalp and hair: Shampoo weekly or fortnightly (but see *Dandruff*).

Face and ears: Face cloth, hot soapy water, twice daily see *Acne*).

The tunnel of the ear should be left alone (for wax in the ears, see under *Deafness*).

Teeth: As in *Halitosis* (2).

Hands: As required; and always after using the lavatory, and before eating.

Arms and Armpits: Once daily.

Feet: Twice a week; daily in summer, and always before swimming in pools.

Bath or shower at least twice a week, ideally once daily. A shower is claimed to be more hygienic as the dirt is washed off and away. On the other hand a hot bath is very relaxing and the objection that one is 'bathing in dilute sewage' can largely be countered by the routine of washing the face before entering, then hands, arms, legs, trunk, genital area (see *Foreskin*), and last, just before getting out, the skin around the anus.

There can be no doubt that present 'toilet' arrangements make soiling of this last mentioned area almost inevitable; a state which will continue until provision of bidets or disposable wet swabs becomes general. In spite of difficulties, every effort should be made to wash genital and anal areas each day.

Underclothes should be changed twice weekly if cotton; daily if nylon, which is much less absorbent.

There are inconsistencies in the present practice of shaving body hair. Most women but few men shave the armpits. The risk of malodour is less if hair is kept shaved. Many women who shave their legs for cosmetic reasons leave the pubic hair intact, yet this is open to contamination by urine and vaginal mucus, and there is a case for considering the adoption of shaving as practised in some tropical communities.

142 Hypothermia

Hypothermia. Old people are bad at regulating their body heat, and in cold conditions their temperature falls far below normal — hypothermia. They are then liable to heart failure or pneumonia. People living alone are most at risk, particularly if they have a fall during the night, and cannot get back into bed, or if through confusion, they don't operate their heating arrangements. An old person who has spent the night out of bed needs a doctor (**UU, U** or **D**, depending on circumstances) as does one whose heating is found to have failed in severe weather. Meanwhile, they should be well, but not heavily, wrapped, and given frequent small hot drinks, if conscious and able to swallow. Whatever can be done to heat the room should be done, but hot water bottles or electric blankets must not be used. (See *Exposure*)

Hysterectomy. The womb (uterus) resembles a medium-sized carrot. At the end of a pregnancy it has grown to a 10-lb. bag; and that more closely represents its place in one's emotional consciousness, and the sense of loss at its removal — which is what the operation of hysterectomy means. To a woman of child-bearing age, the loss of the uterus is a serious, even calamitous thing, and she will need every help and comfort that can be given her. Some older women experience emotional disturbance which cannot be explained by the mechanics of a comparatively simple operation, and which may arise partly from the patient's constitution, partly from remembered folklore, and foolish gossip; and perhaps from the finality of realizing that the reproductive phase of life is over.

The need for hysterectomy more often arises after childbearing is over, usually for the treatment of excessive or irregular *menstruation* or bleeding after the *menopause,* or to prevent the spread of *cancer* of the uterus. To help the diagnosis, the minor operation of dilatation and curettage (known as 'D and C') is often performed first. It needs a short anaesthetic and only a few days in hospital. A common indication for hysterectomy is the presence of *fibroids* — fibrous lumps which form in the muscular walls of the uterus. **They are not cancerous.**

The internal organs of a woman

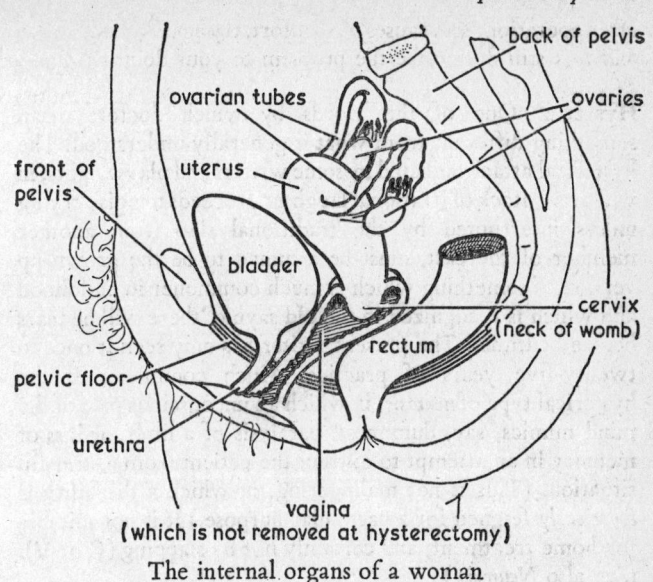

There are two common sequels to the operation:

1 The ovaries often cease to function in the course of the following two or three years, producing symptoms of *menopause* — menstrual loss will of course cease when the uterus is removed (with the rare exception when a remnant of uterine tissue has been left attached to the neck of the womb).
2 The patient may gain weight. The cause of this is not clear, but in some patients it follows increased food intake as a result of emotional disturbance.

Hysterectomy does not usually reduce either the capacity or wish for sexual intercourse, and it is likely that anyone finding otherwise has been bewitched by loose talk. Unless advised otherwise by one's surgeon — and it is perfectly reasonable to ask to speak privately to him before leaving hospital, both about this and the rate of resuming physical work — intercourse can be resumed gently five or six weeks after operation. If it causes discomfort, try again after a week, and if it still does, take the problem to your doctor (C).

Hysteria. One of the words by which doctors mean something different from what is generally understood. The hysterical attack depicted by some writers and playwrights, in which an attack of irrational laughter proceeds to noisy crying unless interrupted by the traditional slap from another member of the cast, must be assumed to be the grown-up version of something which is much commoner in childhood and which is recognized in the old saying 'there will be tears before bedtime'. The present writer has only seen it once in twenty-five years of practice. Much commoner is the hysterical type of *neurosis*, in which an unconscious part of the mind mimics, say, dumbness, paralysis of a limb, or loss of memory in an attempt to extract the patient from a stressful situation. (This is not malingering, in which a disability is *consciously* feigned for a particular purpose.) It is not suitable for home treatment; and certainly not by slapping (C or V). (See also *Neurosis*.)

Immunization (see *Vaccination*).

Impetigo. A crusty infection of the skin, usually on the face and often starting from a crack at the corner of the mouth or at the ear lobe, where germs gain access. The size of the patch slowly increases and the fluid which exudes forms a straw-coloured crust. Infection can be carried to others by contact, and as soon as the condition is recognized, the patient's towel, facecloth, and pillowslip should be boiled, this being repeated each day until he is cured, to prevent him re-infecting himself. Medical advice should be taken, as most cases can be quickly cured by correct treatment (S). Infected children cannot go to school.

Impotence. Failure in the male to achieve the physical requirements of intercourse. It has nothing to do with sterility, which implies failure to conceive following satisfactory intercourse. Although impotence is occasionally due to physical disorder, most cases arise as a by-product of anxiety, psychological illness, or stress. *Anxiety* is responsible for nearly all difficulty of this kind occurring on *honeymoon*. A bridegroom's lack of experience and fear of failure alert primitive defence mechanisms, which (as explained under *Anxiety*) react to insecurity by tensing the body for fight or avoiding action. In the course of establishing these priorities, activities less important for immediate survival are suppressed, and the marital débâcle ensues. Avoidance is by preliminary planning, described under *Honeymoon*. In the confidence of mutual knowledge and understanding, difficulties will be few and of short duration.

A middle-aged man who has had to concentrate energy on his career at the expense of family matters, may run into trouble if the strains of coping with adolescents and his wife's menopause coincide. Recovery often occurs spontaneously if the stresses are lessened, or if the patient is able to readjust his attitude to accommodate them. As there may be an element of treatable depression in the situation, a doctor should be consulted at the onset of trouble (C).

The value now attached to sexual athleticism in fiction may support a belief that normal sexuality involves the wish for, and expectation of, twice nightly intercourse by each partner respectively and indefinitely. Not so; the average, if the word has any value in such a widely varying activity, is to be found at a much less feverish level.

Incontinence. Loss of control of bladder or bowel. There are numerous causes, many of them treatable, all needing medical assessment (C). (See *U and I*).

Incubation Period. The time between exposure of a patient to an infectious disease and his development of the disease. The figures vary in different epidemics, but a broad average is given under the name of each disease.

Indigestion. A vague term not corresponding to any disease. Discomfort lasting for some hours after a meal excessive in quantity or quality might be so described; any more definite or recurring complaint should be the subject of medical advice (C). The simple situation outlined above should be treated with a small teaspoonful of bicarbonate of soda and a few mouthfuls of milk; repeated once only, if necessary, after two or three hours.

Infantile paralysis (see *Poliomyelitis*).

Inflammation. For our purpose, inflammation of the skin or flesh below it, usually caused by entry of *germs* through a breach of the skin's surface (which may be too small to see), occasionally by germs travelling from an infected area elsewhere. The area is painful (often throbbing), hot, red, and swollen. Rest the part, applying *hot bathing* or packs while waiting to attend the doctor (S). *On no account prick or squeeze any inflamed part*; this breaks the barriers which are forming, and spreads infection into the body. If a pale red line is seen wandering up a limb from an inflamed area, such as a *septic finger*, or a tender *lump* forms in the corresponding groin or armpit, the doctor should see it the same day. (Inflammation can also arise from non-bacterial causes such as *gout* and *rheumatism*.)

Influenza. A group of feverish illnesses caused by virus infection. Coming on in the course of a few hours, the patient complains of any, or all, of: sore throat, headache, feverishness, aching limbs and back, nausea and vomiting. The two last are often called gastric influenza, and caused by a virus other than true influenza. The illness is of varying severity, depending on the type of virus, the patient's immunity, and his general state of health. The average uncomplicated case will be feverish and poorly for two or three days, often developing a dry cough which 'loosens' and clears in the course of ten days. Once the temperature has been normal or below for 24–48 hours, the patient can get up, but should not go out of doors for a further two or three days — longer if the weather is bad.

Aspirin or *paracetamol* with *steam inhalations*, and Gee's *Linctus* will make the ordinary attack more bearable, and the doctor is more often called to supply a certificate than for medical help

(V). Complications, such as ear infection (see *Earache*), bronchitis or pneumonia (see under *Cough*), can occur if bacterial infection is implanted on the original virus, usually after four or five days; though there is a rare form of pneumonia which strikes within a few hours of the onset, with collapse and rapid shallow breathing, and calls for urgent medical help (UU).

A late complication is *depression*, lasting for a few weeks after the attack, and sometimes severe (S, occasionally V).

So-called gastric 'flu' ('winter vomiting disease', 'epidemic gastroenteritis') presents as acute *gastritis* and is sometimes associated with a variable degree of diarrhoea. It usually responds to the remedies described for *gastroenteritis* in the course of a few days, but if complicated by *vertigo* may need the doctor's help (D or V). Yearly influenza vaccination in the autumn protects most people to whom it is given.

Injuries. The treatment of minor or local injuries is covered under: *abrasions, cuts, burns, dressings, bleeding, wounds*. All head injuries and those to limbs or trunk sufficient to arouse suspicion of a *fracture* or internal injury, need the early attention of first aid personnel, nurse, or doctor. Meanwhile, interference should be the minimum required to remove patient from danger and to observe the following precautions:

Head injury: 1 If conscious, control any *bleeding*, cover wounds with clean *dressing*. Make the patient comfortable.
2 If unconscious, the power of coughing foreign matter out of the windpipe may be lost, so priority goes to seeing that the airway is clear, and preventing blood, vomit, etc, running into the lungs. Obviously, if blood or saliva is running back from the nose or mouth, the patient must be turned with the face sideways and down until it flows out of the mouth. *If there is suspicion of broken neck or spine, the turning or rolling needs several helpers to ensure that no twisting or bending of the neck or spine occurs.* It should only be attempted if it is vital to prevent suffocation. Pillows or rolled padding should be used to prevent the head flopping as it turns, and head, shoulder, and hip bone should all turn at the same speed. Treatment of bleeding and wounds as for (1).

148 Injuries

Trunk: A moderately severe blow or fall will cause bruising or tearing of the muscles which bind the ribs to each other, and may crack one or more ribs. The patient is temporarily 'winded' but recovers in the course of some minutes, to complain of fairly severe pain each time he breathes, coughs or moves, but does not usually show symptoms such as *shock* or severe shortness of breath. These can follow a more severe injury when the force of the blow carries the fractured rib ends inwardly, causing damage to heart, lungs, spleen, or liver, with collapse, shock, and shortness of breath. In these cases the prevention or treatment of shock is very important (see *Shock*) and transportation to hospital is urgent. The simpler injuries described first usually allow the patient to make his way or be transported to doctor or hospital at a convenient speed and time.

Another form of rib injury is seen in road accidents, when a heavy blow fractures several ribs, with their attached muscles, in two places, so that a 'raft' of muscle-plus-rib bulges out when the patient tries to exhale and prevents air being expelled from the lungs. If the fractured area is large, it can make breathing impossible, and it must be supported by the flat of the hand or a firm pad so that it moves in and out with the rest of the chest as the patient breathes. This support will have to be continued until the patient comes under hospital care. Any puncture wound of the chest, however small, needs medical advice (U or UU if breathing is affected).

Spine: The spine may be injured by direct violence or indirectly, as by a heavy load falling on the bent shoulders, or by the patient falling on the head or heels. Depending on the type and position of injury, a fracture or dislocation, or both, can occur in the neck, thoracic spine (behind the rib cage), or lumbar region. The great, even mortal, danger, is that the spinal cord may be severed either at the time of the injury or by movement of the injured parts subsequently. Except to gain an airway or to remove the patient from imminent danger, no attempt should be made to move a patient who complains of pain or immobility of any part of the back or neck or who cannot move any of his fingers and toes at will, or who cannot feel touching or pinching of the skin of any limb (see above, *Heady injury* (2)). While skilled help is summoned, prevention of *shock* is the first priority. Any considerable bleeding should be controlled with the minimum of disturbance.

Abdomen: It is not safe to assume that a wound of the abdomen, however small, is a triviality; apparently minor wounds may penetrate internally. Such patients should be brought under medical care in the course of two hours (**U**). A blow on the abdomen which does not wound may still so injure an internal organ that it bleeds, and it is safest for all such victims to be seen by their doctor the same day (**S** or **D**). If the patient shows signs of *shock* or complains of pain in either shoulder, the matter is much more urgent (**U** or **UU**).

Pelvis: Severe injury is caused by direct violence or heavy fall. The patient is usually shocked, in severe pain, and feels that his body is coming apart. He may have tried to stand and found that he can't; he should be prevented from moving and also advised not to try to pass water, for the bladder's drainage system may have been damaged. Attend to any bleeding and prevention of *shock*, while waiting for skilled help.

Legs: An older person who falls often fractures the neck (top end) of the thigh bone (femur). The force of the fall may press the broken ends together, so that the joint can still move, although it is painful. If the feet are compared, that on the fractured side may seem to be splayed outwards. If the shaft of the thigh bone is broken, there is swelling and pain at the site, and great pain with the slightest attempt at movement.

Knee: (See also *Knees, Common Disorders*.) Direct violence can produce bruising with or without fracture of the bones surrounding the joint. If pain and bruising are severe, treat as if fractured and prevent patient bearing weight until help arrives.

Lower leg: The common fracture is through both bones (tibia and fibula) which break below and above the middle point of the leg respectively. This fracture is usually obvious from pain, *shock*, swelling, and an obvious angle in the leg, and is also often compound, as the tibia lies close under the skin.

Ankle: If sprained, pain and swelling are to the front of the outer knob of the ankle. If the knob itself is tender, it may be fractured. In the more serious Pott's fracture, the pain and tenderness are worse over the inner knob, and the sole of the foot may be turned outwards. The patient may find that he can hobble on the foot, but should be dissuaded, pending expert assessment.

Treatment of Leg Injuries: Unless obviously minor or trivial, it is wise at first contact to treat as if a fracture were present, and to prevent movement beyond that needed to move the patient from any danger. *Bleeding* should be controlled, wounds dressed (see *Dressing*), and if possible the limb supported with pads and cushions in the position in which it is found. *Shock* is a real hazard in leg fracture, due to internal bleeding, and conservation of heat with blankets, etc, is important. It is probably best to avoid drinks unless it is certain that an anaesthetic will not have to be given in the next few hours. If it becomes necessary to move the patient, the best way of 'splinting' is to tie the legs together in several places, padding above the ankles and above and below the knees (to keep pressure off the bony areas), then to lift as a whole, with several pairs of joined hands, or folded towels, passed under the patient in four or five places. Do not take weight on an injured leg or foot without medical advice.

Upper Limb Injuries: Unless caused by direct violence, usually result from a fall with outstretched arm, the injury occurring at the part which proves weakest at the time of impact.

The **Wrist** may be *sprained* — swollen and painful, or *fractured* (Colles' fracture), when it will appear deformed if viewed from the side, as compared with the uninjured wrist. At the **Elbow**, *dislocation* or fracture both produce great pain, made worse by any attempt at movement (which should not be persisted in). Elbow injury can obstruct a blood vessel, and if forearm or hand is seen to be blue or white it is very urgent to secure medical aid (UU, or immediate transport to hospital casualty department). If the force of injury falls higher up it may fracture the upper end of the arm bone (**Humerus**) a little below the shoulder. Still higher, the **Collar Bone** (felt like a stick of firewood across the top of the chest from breast bone to shoulder) may be fractured.

For all these injuries, having stopped bleeding and dressed any wound, the next step is to support the forearm, including wrist and elbow, in a sling (see illustration, below) and get the patient to doctor or casualty department with precautions against shock.

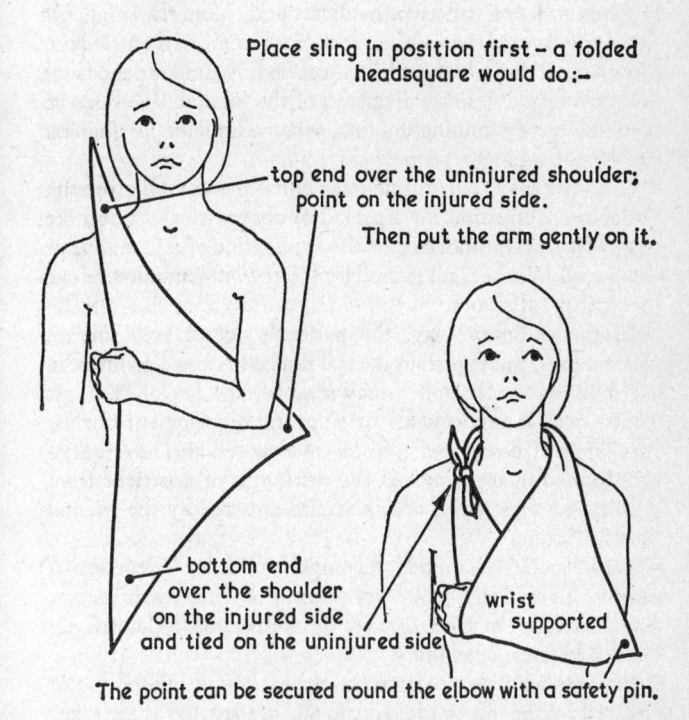

Place sling in position first – a folded headsquare would do:–

top end over the uninjured shoulder; point on the injured side.

Then put the arm gently on it.

bottom end over the shoulder on the injured side and tied on the uninjured side

wrist supported

The point can be secured round the elbow with a safety pin.

Making a sling

Inherited Diseases. Genetic counselling for couples worried about the possibility of their children inheriting diseases which have occurred in their families, is available on reference to a Genetic Advisory Centre through the family doctor:

Insanity. A legalistic term for the severer forms of mental illness. Under the Mental Health Act, 1959, a person suffering from mental illness can be compulsorily admitted to hospital if the interests of his own health or the protection of others require it. Application is made either by the patient's *nearest* relative or by a Social Worker, and is supported by recommendation of two medical practitioners. It allows detention in hospital *for observation*, for not more than 28 days, after which the case must be re-assessed. A similar procedure is followed if a definite diagnosis of the mental illness can be made by the examining doctors, when admission *for treatment* can be for a longer term.

In emergency, when time does not allow compliance with the above, admission for a period of observation of not more than 72 hours is authorized on the application of *any* relative or the Social Worker, supported by the recommendation of one medical practitioner.

In the ordinary way, the patient's doctor will initiate proceedings, but if serious mental illness becomes manifest in a public place, the police may send for the Social Worker. This official is expert in all the rules and requirements for the admission of cases, and will be able to tell the relatives of provisions for applying for the discharge of a patient from hospital to their care, which is also covered by the Mental Health Act.

A patient detained under a compulsory order is deprived of some of his civil rights. A description of those he retains can be found in *Guide to Civil Liberties* by the National Council for Civil Liberties (Penguin).

Patients who are no danger to themselves or others are not covered by the above procedure, and are treated as are other cases of illness by the doctor making application to the appropriate hospital. (See also *Depression, Schizophrenia*.)

Insomnia. Two main forms: **1** Delay in going to sleep and **2** Waking early.

1 Unless it is caused by pain or illness, delay in going to sleep is usually due to failure of the mind to compose itself for rest. Thinking of the day's or tomorrow's difficulties, or worries in general, maintains the body in a state of readiness for action, with tense muscles and high pulse rate, which is the biological result of confronting problems — most of which, in the days when the human race was young, would require violent physical solutions. The original homo sapiens, whose mind we have inherited, reached the end of the day tired by the physical use of his body. Unless his senses warned him of danger, he lay down and slept for the five or six hours needed completely to restore his strength, then began work again. Nowadays, many reach bed after a day spent using their brains, without dispersing the physical tensions of the body which they have aroused. For those who are unable to leave their problems at the office, or who have no office, the following will help. After a comfortably hot bath (about 15 minutes), the patient lies in bed and writes on a piece of paper clipped to a board a list of all the problems encountered during the day, confining the description of each item to three or four words. When complete, the list is gone over from the beginning, and a short note is set against any item which calls for action the next day, the item being marked in the right hand margin. The board is put aside and the patient either composes himself for sleep or reads a book until he feels sleepy. In the morning, the paper is removed and replaced by a blank sheet for that evening. As each marked item is dealt with during the day it is cancelled.

Of course, in the stress of serious events, such methods may not serve for a time, and one's doctor should then be consulted for help in tiding one over into calmer waters. Waking in the small hours of the morning can be caused by external noise, early daylight in summer, the need to pass water, or rheumatic pains, and stiffness. The last often responds satisfactorily to two *aspirins* or *paracetamol* tablets, and the single dose should be put within reach with a small amount of milk to swallow it with, the night before. (See *Night rising*.)

Persistent early morning waking for none of the above reasons is often due to an attack of *depression* and the patient should consult his doctor for advice and treatment (C).

If sedatives are ordered to help with sleep, remember not to leave the container within reach of the bed, as there is a danger of forgetting that one has taken the dose, and taking several more tablets in semi-conscious confusion.

Note: A regular heavy drinker may complain of sleeplessness in general terms. This is one of the warnings that an attack of *delirium* tremens may be on the way, and a strong effort should be made to get him to his doctor (S).

Internal Organs (see illustration on p. 155).

Intoxication. A euphemism for Drunkenness.
Drinking alcohol has two short-term effects:

1 The alcohol is absorbed from the stomach and circulates through the system, acting as a mild anaesthetic, reducing the brain's power of judgement, lengthening reaction time, and impairing the ability to make skilled movements. This is the socially important effect, by reason of its relation to motor transport.
2 The alcohol may irritate the stomach lining and produce acute gastritis, which will begin to make itself felt a few hours later.

Treatment: There is no treatment for (1) except to wait for the excess to be eliminated from the system — usually several hours. A patient who has drunk himself *unconscious* will need admission to hospital, as it may be necessary to use a stomach pump. The worst effects of (2) can be avoided by taking a large teaspoonful of bicarbonate of soda with a glass of water before retiring, and two or three *paracetamol* tablets in the morning.

- **If a patient is not within the scope of home care, or worsens in spite of it, or if there is any uncertainty, a doctor should be consulted.**

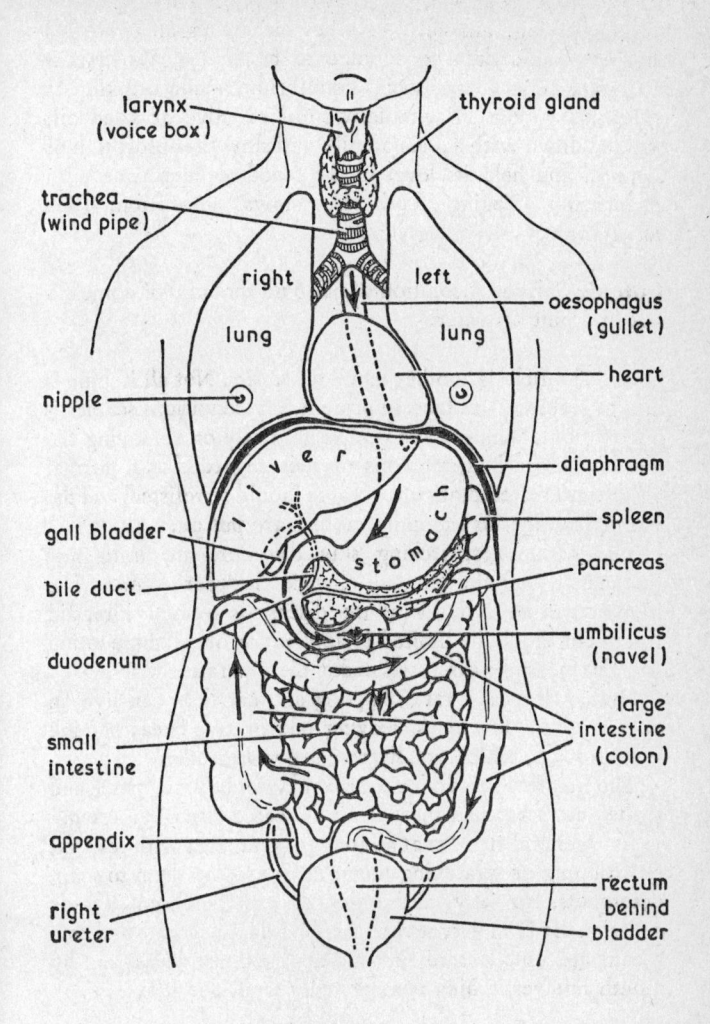

INTERNAL ORGANS
The arrows indicate the direction of movement of the intestinal contents

Prevention: There is no satisfactory combination of alcohol and motor driving, and anyone who anticipates an evening's drinking has a duty to arrange to be driven. When it is necessary to maintain social equilibrium while drinking, a preliminary dose of a tablespoonful of olive or salad oil, washed down with a glass of milk will slow the absorption of alcohol, and help its level in the blood to keep pace with elimination. Taking food also slows absorption. (See *Alcoholism*).

Isotonic Saline. A solution of one 5 ml spoonful of domestic salt in a pint of water.

Itch. 'The Itch' is another name for *scabies*. Not all itching is due to scabies — in fact, in present-day conditions scabies is uncommon. Itching often occurs naturally on removing the clothes before bed, and this may be regarded as a normal reaction. The temptation to scratch should be resisted, and the itching subsides as the night clothes are put on.

The commonest itching skin disorders are *nettle rash* (urticaria) and the related allergic disorder *eczema*. The itching will be relieved as the disease is treated. First aid treatment should be limited to application of calamine lotion and the measures discussed under the separate entries.

Human fleas are rare, but dog and cat fleas can live on humans for a few days, leaving one or two areas of pink itching spots, which usually respond to *hot bathing*.

The first few spots of *chickenpox* may not be recognized, and if they are scratched there is an increased risk of scarring.

As a general rule, treat all itching conditions with respect, not rubbing or scratching them, nor exposing them to soap, detergents, or any antiseptics, until diagnosed. (**S** or occasionally **D** in very severe cases.) Calamine lotion and zinc cream are usually safe first aid applications, and *aspirin* by mouth relieves itching unexpectedly well. See *Lice*.

Jaundice. Yellowing of the skin and whites of the eyes. A condition in which the bile produced by the liver finds its way into the circulation instead of being excreted through the.

bowel. Two frequent causes are infectious hepatitis (catarrhal jaundice) and gallstones. The former is due to a virus infection of the liver and may start with feelings of 'gastric 'flu' — fatigue, feverishness, upper abdominal discomfort, and sometimes vomiting. After some days, the urine is noticed to be dark, the motions pale, and the whites of the eyes yellow when seen in daylight. The colour usually spreads to the whole skin, which may itch. Jaundice from gallstones often follows an attack of severe upper abdominal pain, when a gallstone blocks the bile duct. It is important that the doctor should be able to establish the cause of jaundice (V, keeping a urine specimen) and the pain from gallstone colic needs urgent relief as it is sometimes very severe (U).

Infectious hepatitis is a notifible infectious disease, and the Community Health Department will arrange for a visit to the patient to advise on management. Meanwhile, observe scrupulous toilet precautions, as described under *typhoid fever*.

Kaolin Mixture BNF (British National Formulary). The standard treatment for diarrhoea of recent origin. Two 5 ml spoonfuls taken every four hours until symptoms cease, for an adult. It should not be persisted in after that, as it will reinforce the period of 'constipation' which often lasts a day or two after an attack of diarrhoea. It should not be used for continuing diarrhoea, for which the cause should be ascertained by the doctor.

A special mixture is sold for children, the dose of which is one 5 ml spoonful three times a day for children of one year, two 5 ml spoonfuls for older ones. A child of under one year with diarrhoea should see the doctor (D or S) as should an older child if it does not abate after twenty-four hours, or before that, if the patient is obviously in a bad way.

Kaolin Poultice. Comes in a tin, 250 g or 500 g, and usually has instructions on it. To prepare a first poultice, remove lid and stand the tin in a saucepan of gently boiling water for about a quarter of an hour, mixing slowly with a palette knife or stout piece of stick. When the contents are hot, take a piece of lint of the required size, spoon out some poultice on the smooth side of the lint, and spread it quickly all over to the depth of one-eighth inch. Cover the sticky side with *one layer* of gauze or butter muslin to prevent the poultice sticking to the skin. Now test the sticky side on the back of your hand to be sure that it is not too hot, then apply it to the affected part. Put a pad of cotton wool over all to contain the heat, and support the poultice in any convenient way. Provided it is not soiled by discharge, the same poultice can be reheated once or twice by placing it sticky side up on a plate and steaming it over a saucepan of boiling water. Poultices should be renewed or reheated every two to four hours, depending on circumstances.

Kaolin poultice can be rather messy to deal with, and is most useful for applying to awkward parts of the body where it can be fixed with adhesive plaster. In more accessible parts, *hot bathing, hot packs*, or a guarded *hot water bottle* are more convenient.

Kidney Disease. Roughly of three sorts:

1 Infection in the ureter, the pipe collecting the urine from the kidney and taking it to the bladder. This is **pyelitis**, and often the symptoms are similar to those of *cystitis*, with frequent passage of urine causing a scalding pain. In addition, there may be fever and pain in the loin. In older people pyelitis can produce a state of confusion which masks the true cause (**D, V,** or if mild **S**, taking *specimen of urine*).

2 Pyelitis sometimes complicates the presence of **kidney stone**, but a stone can cause trouble on its own, and if it becomes stuck in the tube, the pain can be very intense, extending from the loin to the groin. This is 'renal colic' and the pain needs the doctor's help for relief (**U**). Meanwhile, a guarded *hot water bottle* to the loin and one or two teaspoonsful of brandy or other spirit every half hour or so will help.

3 **Nephritis**, commoner in children. This is an inflammation of the delicate filtration tissue of the kidney, and usually follows a throat infection by streptococcal germs after about ten days. It is discussed under its own heading.

Knees, Common Disorders of 159

There is a continual need for kidneys for transplantation into patients whose own kidneys are too diseased to work properly. Anyone willing that their kidneys should be so used after their death should complete and carry a Kidney Donor Card — usually available from the family doctor.

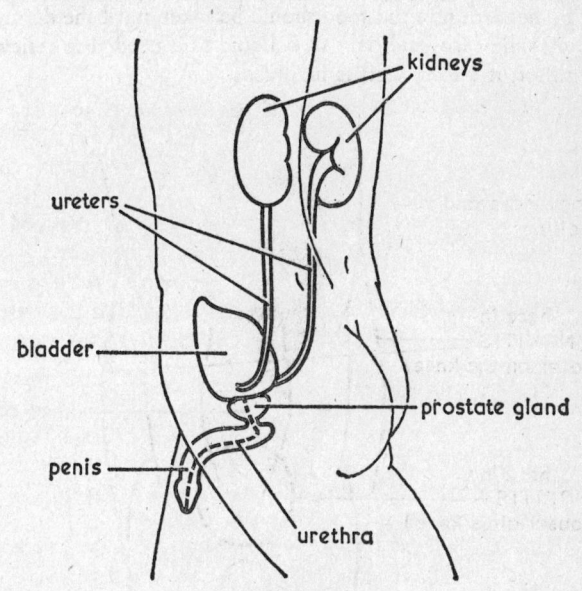

The urinary organs of a man

Knees, Common Disorders of.
1 Housemaid's knee (see under that heading).
2 Water on the knee ('Synovitis'). Formation of fluid in the joint, usually following an injury, and seen as a swelling of the whole joint when viewed from the front and compared with the other knee. *Treatment:* Rest the leg with knee straight on cushions or a pillow. The whole length of the leg from heel to thigh must be supported (**V**). This applies to serious cases. Mild cases can safely be driven to the doctor's surgery (**S**).
3 Locking of the knee joint, due to jamming of a split

160 Knees, Common Disorders of

cartilage. The knee is fixed in one position, usually after a fall with a twist, and attempts to move it are very painful. Treat with *aspirin* or *paracetamol*. Get leg into comfortable position with support of cushions and ask doctor to call (D), or transport patient to hospital. As an anaesthetic may be needed, no solid food should be taken until the doctor sees the case, and only such liquid as is needed to relieve thirst, if a long wait is involved.

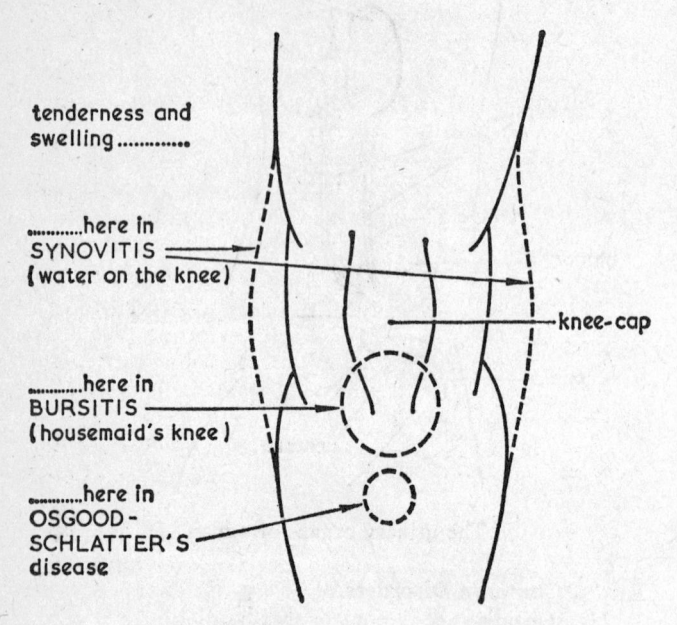

tenderness and swelling..............

..........here in SYNOVITIS (water on the knee)

knee-cap

..........here in BURSITIS (housemaid's knee)

..........here in OSGOOD-SCHLATTER'S disease

The knee seen from the front (See also p. 140)

4 In some adolescents, the knob of bone about two inches below the knee-cap becomes enlarged and tender. This is due to Osgood-Schlatter's disease, a condition of growing bone which rights itself in the course of time. The doctor should be consulted (C) and some restriction of games and kneeling may be needed for a period of months — sometimes longer.

5 In some younger children the tendency to develop 'knock knee' can be recognized and prevented. It is one of the causes of 'aching legs' complained of after walking. (But see also under *Rheumatic fever* — subacute rheumatism.) When the knees are brought together with the legs straight, the ankles are found to be separate. This is accompanied by inward angulation at the ankle joints, and if that is corrected by the provision of properly wedged heels, and shoes which support the whole foot, the legs will straighten as the child grows. The doctor's advice should be taken (C) as soon as the trouble is noticed. Children wearing wedged shoes *must* attend their doctor regularly for supervision.

It should be mentioned that paragraph (5) represents the writer's own view, and that another school of thought holds that the condition will right itself in time without treatment. If wedged shoes are adopted on medical advice, good results can only be expected if they are worn for all purposes. The child should step out of bed into them in the morning and out of them into bath or bed at night. The situation can be difficult is summer, particularly on the beach, but it is worth persevering.

6 Stiff, aching, painful knees in older people, due to rheumatism either of the soft tissues surrounding the joints, or to osteoarthritis in the joint (see under *Arthritis*) (C).

Labour. The process of producing a child, starting after a *pregnancy* lasting some 40 weeks.

Three 'stages' of labour are recognized.

The First Stage, from the start until the neck of the womb (cervix) is fully open. In a first labour, this may take 10 or 12 hours, but is often less, and may only last an hour or two in subsequent labours.

The Second Stage lasts from the time the mother starts to push the baby out of the opened womb until it is born, and this takes one or two hours — longer for first babies, shorter for others.

The Third Stage is spent waiting for the expulsion of the

'afterbirth'; that is, the placenta, a spongy organ through which the baby's nourishment has passed during pregnancy. This takes from a few minutes to half an hour.

In a first pregnancy, there may be doubt as to whether what is happening *is* the onset of labour. Labour contractions are usually first felt low in the back, sometimes at the bottom of the abdomen. They occur every 20 to 30 minutes at first, lasting from 10 to 30 seconds. The interval between contractions lessens as their duration increases. A sign of the onset of labour may be the 'show' — the passage of pink or red jelly from the vagina.

Occasionally, the first sign of labour is a sudden loss of watery fluid from the vagina. If this happens, apply a pad and lie down, having sent for the ambulance (if booked for hospital) or midwife (for a home confinement). The

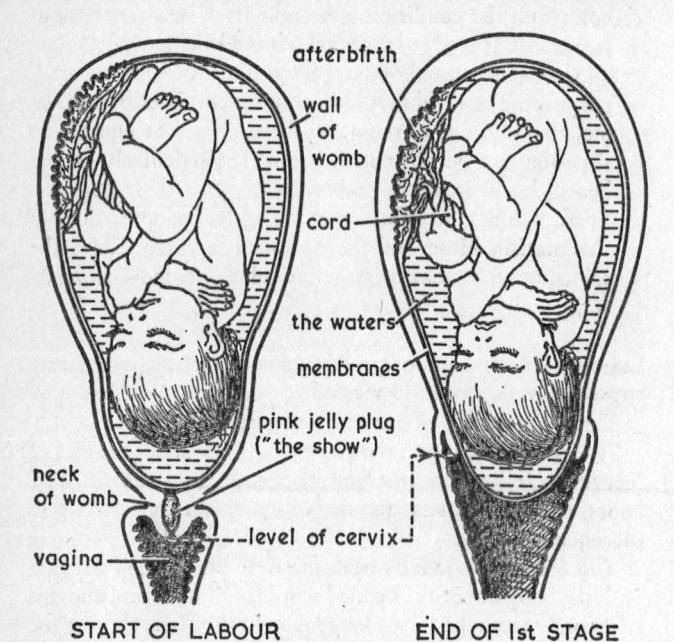

START OF LABOUR   END OF 1st STAGE

The first stage of labour

commonest cause of confusion is with the colic of an attack of *enteritis* though here, the onset of diarrhoea will show what is happening. Occasionally labour may be started by such an attack, and if there is doubt the midwife or doctor should be notified.

When it is clear that labour has started, word should be sent to the midwife or doctor (whichever is conducting the confinement), giving details and time of onset. If the patient is booked for hospital confinement, transport should be summoned. In the first labour, there is no great hurry for this, unless the contractions increase rapidly in force and frequency, occurring every five minutes or so. In subsequent labours there may not be so much time to play with, and it is well to make a move. Early in the first stage the mother may walk about or rest, as she prefers. If resting in a chair or on a bed, she should practise the *relaxation* or breathing routine she has learnt during *pregnancy*. As the first stage proceeds, she may feel more comfortable in bed.

Laxative (see *Aperient, Constipation*).

Lice. Parasites of the hairy areas, where they thrive if undisturbed. In campaign conditions of impaired hygiene, they are sought for at regular inspections. In the absence of these, they set up jungle communities in the hair of the head (head lice), body (body lice), or pubic area (crab lice). They cause itching, and a close search reveals that what had been taken for small flecks of dandruff are really louse eggs (nits), like minute rice grains, each cemented to a hair. Keenly pursuing, one may be rewarded by the sight of an actual louse (lobster- or crab-shaped, about a quarter of an inch long) making for the undergrowth. When the excitement has subsided, the patient should attend the doctor, or clinic.

Linctus. A preparation for easing cough. A useful one can be bought as Gee's Linctus (Squill Opiate Linctus BPC). *It should not be used if patient is seriously ill or if breathing is rapid or difficult.* An otherwise healthy adult can take one or two 5 ml teaspoonfuls up to four times in 24 hours, in a little hot water if the cough is hard or dry. For children, a special strength is sold with dosage directions.

Loss of Voice. Most often due to simple laryngitis (inflammation of the voice box) as a complication of a common cold. If so, it will clear up in a few days if the voice is rested, and *steam inhalations* may be found comforting, every four hours. See a doctor (S), if the voice does not recover in a week or so, to exclude more serious conditions.

Lumbago. Pain in the hollow at the lower end of the back. It is not a disease, but the name of a pain for which there are many causes. Often confused with pain in a kidney, which is usually one-sided and higher up, under the lowest rib. Both kinds of pain can extend downwards, but kidney pain usually travels down to the groin, while lumbago may extend to the buttock and the back of the leg. The most frequent cause of mild lumbago is strain of one of the back muscles or ligaments. It is often not bad enough to keep the patient off work and may clear up in a week or so with the help of *paracetamol* or *aspirin* and a guarded *hot water bottle* to the back at night. During an attack, and for a few weeks after, the power of the strong muscles of the back will be lessened, so that if a strain is thrown on the back, such as by trying to lift with it bent, the whole force of the load may fall on the bones of the spine without protection from the muscles, forcing one of the soft shock-absorber discs out of shape. A mild attack will then be converted into a severe one; the patient may with difficulty get himself upright, or may have to crawl on all fours and half climb, half roll himself on to his bed. He should lie flat on his back on as firm a mattress as possible, supported underneath by boards; a folded bath towel is thrust under his lower back to support it in its natural hollow shape, and he should take *aspirin* or *paracetamol* to relieve pain. He will usually need medical help in the course of the first 24 hours (D or V). If the disc has been pushed against one of the nerves coming from the spinal cord, the pain will be felt down the back of one leg, constituting an attack of sciatica.

A disc prolapse as described above can occur without the

warning of a milder attack, and such should be suspected if pain is severe, extends to the back of the leg, is worse on coughing, and if movement of the back is made impossible by pain.

The victim of a prolapsed lumbar disc is for some years at risk of further attacks, and particular care should be taken against the effects of cold, fatigue, and weakness after infections. The man who returns home with a cold after a tiring day's work to find the coal scuttle empty is inviting trouble if he goes straight out to the coal bunker to refill it.

Ideal sitting position. A tall, high-seated, straight backed chair, with padding in the angle to support the lumbar region. The seat should be high, and short front-to-back, to allow the occupant to stand straight up out of it without bending the lower back. Comfortable conversion of an old wooden chair is usually possible with foam rubber.

A booklet *Lumbar Disc Disorders* is issued free by the Arthritis and Rheumatism Council (see *Arthritis*), but is only obtainable through one's doctor. (See *Backache*.)

Lump. There is one thing to do when a lump is found anywhere in or on the body. Take it to your doctor (S). Most of them are harmless cysts, glands, fatty tumours, etc, but a few are the first sign of cancer, and early recognition can offer the chance of cure.

Lung Cancer and Smoking. Recovery from cancer of the lung can occur after treatment, but it happens sufficiently seldom to make this a very good disease not to have. In round figures, for every non-smoker who dies of lung cancer, 7 men who have smoked up to 15 cigarettes a day and 20 who have smoked up to 30 a day will die. From present knowledge, it appears that cigarette smoking is a main cause, and that it exerts its greatest effect after it has been continued for some 20 years; but there is no level of complete safety. Stopping smoking will reduce the risk of developing the disease. A man who stopped smoking 5 years ago is only half as likely to develop it as one who did not. After 10 years the risk is only one-third.

Although these figures refer to men, among whom the disease is at present more frequent, such figures as are available suggest that women smokers are similarly at risk, though to a less extent.

Magnesium Trisilicate. Best bought from the chemist as compound magnesium trisilicate powder. One or two ounces (25 or 50 grams) may be kept in a stoppered jar safely for many months. For use in acute stomach upsets, half a 5 ml spoonful with a little milk-and-water (equal parts), may be repeated after two hours, and thereafter four hourly.

Note that this is a treatment for *stomach* upset. The powder is too laxative to help an attack of diarrhoea. If tablets are preferred, they can be bought as magnesium trisilicate compound tablets, and the dose is 1 or 2 every four hours. They should be crushed and taken as a powder, or well chewed before swallowing.

Malaria. Travellers to North Africa, Eastern Mediterranean and beyond, should seek advice about protection from malaria (C). Usually, preventive treatment should start before leaving, and continue for a month after return.

Marriage. Anyone approaching marriage and needing information should read *Getting Married*, from Family Doctor Publications, BMA House, Tavistock Square, London, WC1H 9JP, and *Treat Yourself to Sex — A Guide for Good Living*, by Brown and Faulder, published by Dent, and sponsored by the Marriage Guidance Council.

Marriage Guidance. Apply to the National Marriage Guidance Council, Herbert Gray College, Little Church Street, Rugby CV21 3AP, or the Scottish Marriage Guidance Council, 58 Palmerston Place, Edinburgh, EH12 5AZ, for the address of one's nearest local Marriage Guidance Council, if this cannot be found in the local telephone directory. (Send a stamped addressed envelope.)

Masturbation. Pleasurable manipulation of the sex organs. It is often practised by young children of both sexes, forming a natural phase of their development, which they abandon as their outside interests widen. It does no harm and does not call for prevention or disapproval. Masturbation usually recommences in early adolescence, more frequently by boys, and is a harmless result of the flowering of sexual development. Harmless, that is, unless it is made the subject of condemnation and threats of evil results. Worry over masturbation is a constituent of some forms of *neurosis*.

J. D. Hadfield claimed that excessive masturbation could hinder the development of a mature pattern of sexuality, by concentrating the experience of pleasure on oneself, rather than sharing it with somebody else. However, the harm caused by repression of the activity, or by rebuke, is the greater.

If a child is conscious of love and affection, and if his developing curiosity is matched by increasing outside interests, the problem of excess should not arise.

Measles. One of the common infectious disorders, usually experienced in childhood. Typically, after a stubborn dry cough has lasted three or four days (and nights!), an irregular blotchy rash develops on neck and face and spreads down over the whole body. The patient is feverish, occasionally severely ill, and the cough is uncontrollable for a few days. The onset resembles a severe cold affecting nose and eyes, and the eyes may hurt when exposed to bright light. For this reason only, the windows can be temporarily shaded, but there is no need to keep the patient in the dark, and light will not physically harm the eyes.

Measles is notifiable, and the doctor should be told (V) when the rash appears, unless he is already in attendance. *Steam inhalations, linctus,* and *blackcurrant tea* are useful.

Immunization against measles is now available through the National Health Service, by one injection given during the second year of life.

Incubation: 10–15 days.

Quarantine: 14 days after the appearance of the rash in the patient but children over 5 years are not usually excluded from school.

Medic-Alert. A non-profit making foundation of world-wide extent providing engraved warning bracelets for wear by diabetics, epileptics, and others, so that information can be available to those treating them should they be rendered unconscious by accident or illness.

Particular conditions listed are: Bleeding tendency, immunized against tetanus by vaccine, myasthenia gravis, allergy to penicillin, taking anticoagulants or steroids, allergy to bee stings, wearing contact lenses, diabetes, deaf mute, epilepsy, and others can be added.

The London address is: Medic-Alert Foundation, 9 Hanover Street, London W1R 9HF, and a stamped addressed envelope should be enclosed when writing for details of membership.

Meningitis and **Meningism.** Inflammation of the membranes sheathing the brain and spinal cord. This results in the picture of 'meningism'; severe headache, resentment of light, nausea and/or vomiting, and pain felt in the neck and spine on bending the head forward. Meningism can be secondary to infection elsewhere — commonly to pneumonia in children — and a mild form is often a feature of general virus illness of influenzal type. The term meningitis implies that the sheathing membranes are themselves infected, either by virus, as in 'aseptic meningitis' and *poliomyelitis*, or by bacteria, as in *cerebrospinal meningitis*. The sorting out of the cause of meningism may be complicated, and the doctor should see a case the same day as it starts; give details of the case when calling the doctor, and keep the patient resting until he comes.

Menopause. Usually in the late forties or early fifties menstruation stops. During the last year, the 'period' may skip one or two months, resuming at a calculated date, and behaving as a normal period. Should it be irregular in timing or duration, medical advice should be taken (**C**), as also if a loss, however small, occurs more than six months after the last period. Although most women pass through this phase with only minor alterations in mood, it is a time when the psychological balance is less easily maintained than usual, and calls for sympathetic consideration by the family when they become aware of the situation. 'Hot flushes' are not uncommon, and may range from an inconvenience to a major embarrassment. The doctor can usually help with these. The menopause is also a time when *depression* may be experienced, and medical advice should always be sought for this, by the patient herself or by her family if depression is severe or alters sharply in depth. (See also *Shoplifting*.)

While restraint will be required from the husband in the presence of emotional disturbance, as at any other time of crisis, there is no sudden alteration of sexual feelings as a direct result of the menopause, and marital intercourse continues for many years. Medical help may be needed for dryness of the vagina, which may cause discomfort. It is due to reduced hormone production; this brings me to the controversial subject of Hormone Replacement Therapy (HRT). If I may attempt a balanced view, it is that a majority of doctors in the United Kingdom would prescribe hormone replacement (in tablet form) for the treatment of symptoms attributable to hormone deficiency after the menopause, who might not all be happy to continue long-term hormone therapy in the absence of symptoms. This leaves unsolved the problem of post-menopausal calcium loss from the bones, which can become more liable to fracture, and on the other hand, the possibility of adverse effect from long-term hormone treatment.

Menstruation. Usually starts in the twelfth to fourteenth year and lasts until the late forties or early fifties. With fairly wide variations, the onset is usually at monthly intervals and duration three to five days. It is a natural process and represents the shedding of the soft lining specially laid down in the womb for reception of an egg, should the latter become fertilized. An egg is usually expelled from the ovary ('ovulation') about halfway between two menstrual 'periods' and makes its way into the womb through one of the two ovarian tubes. If it encounters a sperm introduced during sexual intercourse, the first stage of a pregnancy has commenced, and the fertilized egg settles in the soft 'nesting' lining of the womb which is prepared afresh for each egg. If the egg is not fertilized, this lining is not needed, and is shed about two weeks after ovulation, appearing as a brown/red discharge from the vagina. This is not 'bleeding' in the true sense of the word; if it becomes so it needs medical aid (see *Bleeding from the womb*), but the discharged tissues contain a good deal of haemoglobin, the raw material of red blood corpuscles, and consequently women often have a marginal degree of *anaemia* during the reproductive period of life, which may need correction by taking iron. Before the onset of regular menstruation, girls may experience a variable amount of discomfort in the lower abdomen, and this may be difficult to distinguish from other causes of pain. The first few 'periods' may not be regular in their interval, but once regularity is established, any marked irregularity of time, duration, or quantity should be reported to the doctor (C), and so should bleeding after intercourse.

Painful menstruation is not natural, and much of it is caused by nervous tension, often the result of primitive ideas, and failure to arm the girl beforehand with an unemotional account of what she may expect, and its significance. Occasionally pain is due to physical causes and then needs medical or surgical treatment (S). A 'painful period' at a time of nervous stress will respond to a few hours resting in bed with a guarded *hot water bottle* to the abdomen and another to the soles of the feet, having taken 2 or 3 *aspirin* or *paracetamol* tablets. If constipated, a dose of Epsom or effervescent salts (see *Aperient*) each morning on waking for the rest of the period. This is for the *occasional* occurrence only. *Regularly* painful periods need the doctor's advice.

Some women experience discomfort for a few hours, sometimes with a transient red discharge, about midway between the periods. It is caused by the process of ovulation and is not of serious significance. The discomfort responds to *aspirin* or *paracetamol*.

Failure to menstruate may be due to *pregnancy*, worry, shock (as from sudden bad news), illness or change of routine, as when travelling.

Premenstrual tension is experienced by many women in the week before the menstrual flow. It is associated with retention of fluid in the system, and may give rise to depression, shortness of temper, and headaches. Most cases can be helped by medical treatment (C).

Migraine (Sick Headache). Starts with pain in one side of the head, sometimes with preliminary loss of half the field of vision, or the appearance of coloured zig-zag figures. The pain becomes more severe, often causing prostration, until vomiting occurs, after which it usually clears. Attacks last for four to 24 hours and there may be limpness for a day after a severe one. The name 'bilious attack' came from the appearance of yellow bile in the vomit, and in children the vomiting may overshadow the headache. There is often a family tendency to migraine, and a patient may at times become more prone to attacks, so that they happen in clusters, several in a few weeks, followed by some weeks or months of freedom. Attacks can be caused by unwise eating or drinking, particularly chocolate and pork, and when the patient is tired. Other causes are worry, frustration and hormone troubles; and those with a tendency to 'fibrositis', disc trouble, or rheumatism in the neck (see *Spondylosis*) can develop attacks after using too many pillows or lying in a draught.

Prevention and treatment: The avoidance of known causes, increased *relaxation* and tranquillity, together with such wisdom as comes with the passing of years, are probably responsible for the lessening of attacks as one gets older. A lot can be done both to treat the attacks and lessen their frequency, and the doctor should be consulted (C). Long-term treatment is well worth continuing, if advised.

Home treatment of an attack: Rest in a shaded room, with a *cold pack* over the eyes and temples, and a *hot water bottle* to the feet. Three *aspirin* or *paracetamol* tablets, crushed, taken as early as possible in the attack. Some find that if they can produce vomiting by tickling the back of the throat the attack abates more quickly.

For anyone developing an acute attack of migraine while in London, the Princess Margaret Migraine Clinic now based at Charing Cross Hospital, Fulham Palace Road, London, W.6, provides an 'acute headache' clinic twenty-four hours a day. (Telephone first to make sure.)

Miscarriage. The popular name for what is medically and legally called *abortion*. The victim of a miscarriage who hears the latter term used in a medical discussion (as when a doctor telephones the hospital to arrange treatment) must not assume that anything other than a natural mishap is implied — miscarriage resulting from illegal interference with a pregnancy is called criminal abortion.

In a typical case, after two or three periods have been missed, and often at a time when a period would have occurred, a loss of blood is noticed. It varies from very little to quite a lot, and may be accompanied or followed by spasmodic pain low in the abdomen. What happens next depends on the amount of loss. If this is less than a usual period, the patient should take herself to bed or, if she has the care of children, lie down on a couch, having sent a message to her doctor asking for a call, and stating the time of onset and amount of loss in the above terms. If the loss is heavy or pain is severe, the doctor should be asked to call as soon as possible. The patient is kept warm, and given a warm drink, repeated as required. The ideal companion is someone of suitable temperament who has herself experienced a miscarriage. Any matter passed should be kept in a bowl or other receptacle until the doctor can see it — for this reason the use of a chamber pot is preferred to a WC. Sometimes the complete baby (very small, one to two inches), called the fetus, will be passed in a sudden spasm with, or without, its surrounding membranes, etc. If so, the pain and bleeding will almost cease. Otherwise, after a few days rest the bleeding may stop, and the pregnancy proceed normally. In a few cases the fetus dies at the onset of trouble, but is not discharged and has later to be removed by a minor operation. If bleeding continues in a desultory way for a week or so, the doctor may advise that the patient enters hospital for a curettage, so that blood loss is stopped and the womb cleared out to make ready for another and more successful pregnancy. This is not a serious operation and is performed under a short general anaesthetic.

Aftercare. To suffer a miscarriage is a more distressing experience than is usually understood. Those about the patient should avoid attempts at 'cheering her up', allowing her a few days of sympathetic attention and help to overcome her distress. At this time the relationship between husband and wife, and parents and other child or children, calls for a maximum effort of understanding, and as the husband is usually less affected than the others, the brunt of the effort falls on him. He should practise all the small attentions of courtship and should temporarily abandon outside engagements not immediately required by his work. An only child is particularly vulnerable at this time and every effort should be made to keep him integrated with the parents; avoiding, unless it is impossible, the temptation to let him go and stay with friends or relatives to be out of the way (it may not be put like that, but it will mean that). If there is more than one child, and their relationship with each other is good, then for them both to stay a week or so with trusted and liked grandparents or other close relatives may be a good thing, and will allow husband and wife to concentrate their care and affection on each other while time begins to play its part.

Unless advised otherwise, intercourse can be resumed about four weeks after an abortion or curettage.

Moles. Skin blemishes which take many forms. Most are harmless, though removal may be desired for cosmetic reasons. Removal of a mole is a surgical operation and should only be undertaken by a medical man. Attempts by amateurs often lead to infection or to permanent scarring.

Flattened dark moles are important, as they can occasionally increase in size and set up growth in other parts of the body. The risk is a small but real one, and anyone who has one of these moles which starts to grow should take medical advice at once (S), as also about any dark moles situated on the palm or sole, as some of these are best removed before they give trouble (C).

Morning Sickness (see *Pregnancy*).

174 Motorist's Leg

Motorist's Leg. A painful 'knotted' feeling of the shin muscles developing in the course of a long drive. Several factors are probably involved:

1 The accelerator connections are stiff, needing lubrication.
2 The driving posture is wrong, so that the foot has to be flexed further back than its natural position. Adjustment to the position and rake of the seat should allow the thigh to be supported and the knee and ankle more extended. Note that an 'organ' pedal is not necessarily the best for everyone, as its angle dictates the resting angle of the foot.
3 The muscles concerned are those which lift the foot off the accelerator pedal. A driver facing a long run may be driving faster than he is accustomed, and this leads him to alert the right foot for braking by keeping the withdrawing muscles in play. (See also *Relaxation* (2).)

Treat with *hot packs, aspirin* or *paracetamol*. It usually settles within a few hours. (**S** or **V** if severe or increasing.)

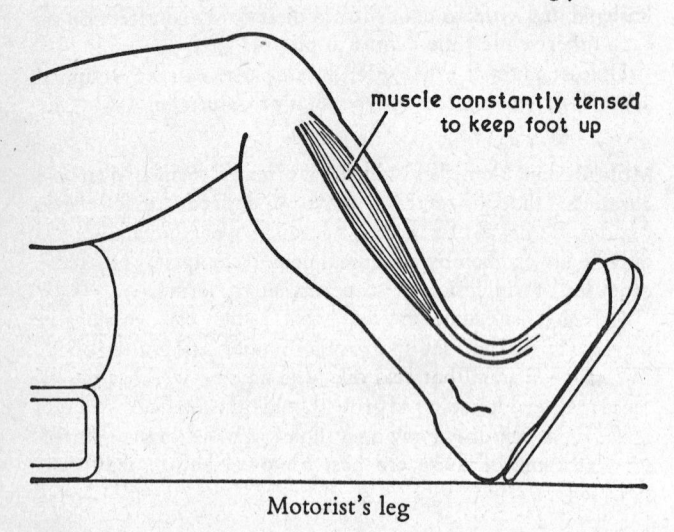

muscle constantly tensed to keep foot up

Motorist's leg

Multiple Sclerosis (mentioned briefly under *'Nerves'*).

Mumps. An inflammation of the salivary glands, usually those of horseshoe shape in front of, below, and behind the lobes of the ears. It is not a notifiable disease and the milder cases clear up without incident if the patient rests in bed until the swelling has completely gone. *Aspirin* may be needed for the first few days and *hot packs* are comforting to the enlarged glands. Appetizing foods and citrus fruits, which will stimulate the inflamed glands, should be avoided at first. The commonest complications, usually in adolescents or adults, are inflammation of the breasts (mastitis) and testicles (orchitis). These call for medical advice (V). A patient is usually regarded as infectious for seven days after all swelling has gone.

A man may reasonably worry after an attack of orchitis, lest it has left him sterile. This does occasionally happen after severe infection of both testicles, but is very rare. Usually, fertility is unaffected.

Incubation: 12 to 24 days.

Quarantine: About 30 days, but usually contacts need not be excluded from school.

Mushroom Poisoning. Mushrooms are not poisonous. If illness follows their consumption, they were not mushrooms. (See *Toadstool Poisoning*. **Urgently**.)
Note: The rare case of allergy to mushroom will produce symptoms of acute *gastroenteritis* and/or *nettle rash*, and should come under medical care urgently, just as if it were toadstool poisoning.

Nails, Common Disorders of.
Ingrowing Toenail. Usually affects the big toe and is most troublesome when it does so. It often results from faulty trimming of the toenails, which should be cut straight across to keep the growing corners clear of the flesh (a). A curved cut results in these corners digging into the flesh (b), as the nail grows; the invaded area of the toe then becomes septic. Once this has happened the doctor should be consulted (C).

While waiting to see him, bathing with hot *normal saline* for five to ten minutes every four hours will relieve discomfort. If there is no inflammation and the nail corners have not penetrated the skin, the situation can often be saved by cleansing with warm soapy water each night, after which the skin folds are gently pushed clear of the advancing nail corners with a clean orange stick. This is continued nightly until the growing corners reach the end of the toe, when the nail can be cut straight across, leaving the trimmed nail as shown in (a).

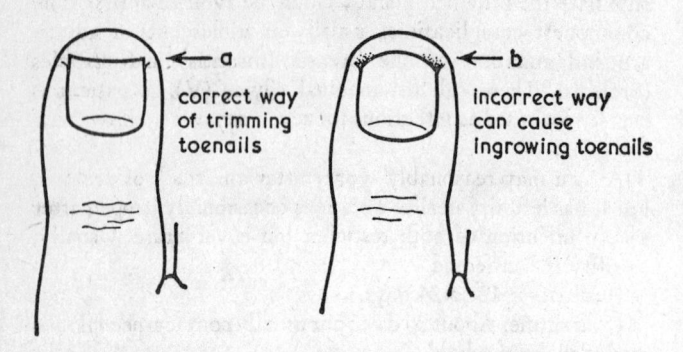

← a correct way of trimming toenails

← b incorrect way can cause ingrowing toenails

Bruising, by a blow, results in a blood blister which forces the nail away from its bed and is acutely painful. Rather than suffer this, it is worth attending hospital casualty department or doctor (S), as the pressure can be relieved by painlessly puncturing the nail with a drill or hot wire.

Infection of the nail fold, called paronychia. This is dealt with under *Finger, poisoned.*

Flaking and breaking of fingernails. Seems to happen more often to women, and contact with detergents and similar substances has been blamed. Whether or not this is just, it seems sensible to protect the nails with rubber or plastic gloves, and to wear work gloves for household chores. Improvement has been reported after eating two grams of gelatine *daily for 3 or 4 months* — that is, a generous 5 ml spoonful of powdered gelatine, or quarter of a pint jelly, either straight from the packet or prepared (any flavour).

Proteinized applications are now on the market (through pharmacists) which are intended to have the same effect by direct application to the nails. Any treatment used must be continued for many weeks, without intermission, as all are intended to strengthen the new nail substance as it is formed.

Napkin Rash. Damage to the skin of a baby by exposure to urine. Some of the worst cases occur when the nappy contains bacteria left behind from a previous bowel action. These are not destroyed by ordinary napkin washing and when urine is passed into such a contaminated nappy, it is fermented by the bacteria, releasing ammonia, which causes a chemical burn of the skin. If the baby is teething, or is feverish for any reason, a more concentrated and more damaging urine is passed, and it is more than ever necessary to change wet nappies promptly. The longer and closer the contact, the worse the effects, and the use of waterproof knickers for any but short-term social convenience should be avoided. Disposable napkins limit bacterial contamination, and 'one-way' nappies reduce contact irritation.

The usual appearance is of a patchy red rash, sometimes with a brownish tinge. If the skin is sensitive, or moist conditions occur inside plastic knickers, a weepy eczema may quickly arise, and this can spread to other parts of the body. A variation met with is the occurrence of separate soft blisters over the napkin area. Any but mild cases should have medical advice (C). Otherwise, exposure to warm air as much as possible, cleansing with warm *isotonic saline* (not soap and water) and use of a zinc cream, will allow healing to take place, provided napkins are boiled between each application or disinfected in one of the special solutions available from the chemist.

Nephritis. Inflammation of the kidneys which results in their being unable to filter and eliminate unwanted matter from the system. Not to be confused with *pyelitis* in which the inflammation is in the drainage tube leading from the kidney to the bladder.

- **If a patient is not within the scope of home care, or worsens in spite of it, or if there is any uncertainty, a doctor should be consulted.**

Acute nephritis usually starts a week or two after an attack of septic throat or tonsillitis. The first sign may be a considerable reduction in the amount of urine passed — none at all in severe cases. The salt and fluid not eliminated cause waterlogging of the body, so that by evening the ankles and feet may be swollen. When the patient lies down, the fluid drains out of the legs and causes puffiness of the face and eyelids, visible in the morning. This appearance in a child should prompt inquiry as to how much water has been passed in the previous 24 hours, and the doctor should be informed (D). Meanwhile, the patient rests in bed taking the *least* amount of water and glucose (1 or 2 teaspoons in half a pint) flavoured with lemon or orange juice, that will prevent thirst; and no solid foods. No attempt should be made to 'flush out the system' as this will increase the load on the already damaged kidneys and lessen their chance of recovery.

Most cases recover completely, though hospital care and complicated tests lasting many weeks may be called for.

Acute nephritis is commoner in the young, chronic nephritis in adults. The latter may result from the occasional case of acute nephritis which does not recover completely, or from a variety of causes, one of which is the prolonged use of pain-relieving tablets. The effect of chronic nephritis is to reduce the concentrating power of the kidneys, so that they have to produce a greater amount of more dilute urine and cannot reduce output during the night, as they normally do. Consequently the patient finds him or herself having to pass water one or more times a night, and the appearance of this symptom calls for early investigation (C).

'Nerves'. Another of the words with two meanings. By nerves, doctors mean the bundles of conducting threads which carry information from sense organs to the brain, and commands from the brain to the muscles of the limbs, etc. The communication network, together with the brain and spinal cord, is called the 'nervous system', and a special part of it, the autonomic nervous system, works constantly without our being aware of it, adjusting our intake of air, speed of blood circulation, body temperature, digestion, and concentration of hormones (powerful regulators released into the circulation by the endocrine *glands*) in the system.

Thus a 'nerve doctor' is really a neurologist, dealing with disease of any of the parts of the nervous system, though many will understand the term to imply a psychiatrist, one who deals with disorders and diseases of the mind — that part of the brain of whose working we are aware or can become aware. The two specialities might be thought to overlap, for clearly if something is wrong with the mind, something must in turn be wrong with that part of the brain which provides its mechanism; and this is true, though to a small extent, for in the main, the presumed structural, mechanical, or chemical disorders responsible for trouble in the mind are so minute that they are not accessible to our present methods of neurological investigation. The person who knows most about what is going on in a mind is the person in whose head the mind is, though he may not be able to interpret it. It is the psychiatrist's task by asking questions to build up from the patient's answers a pattern of his mental activity, and to deduce from this the kind of disorder from which he is suffering. (In the same way, when a doctor suspects that a patient has a gastric ulcer, he may be able to deduce its position in the stomach from the patient's reply to questions about the time of onset of pain, its duration, and the effect of food on it.) This is the diagnosis of mental illness, which can vary in severity and curability from the very mild to the very severe. It is often called nervous illness (as in 'nervous breakdown') from a wish to avoid frightening a patient unnecessarily by the suggestion of mental illness.

True nervous illnesses or diseases are such as neuritis, from injury or infection of a nerve; *neuralgia* from disorder of a sensory nerve bundle; multiple sclerosis, a scarring of various parts of the brain and spinal cord, putting some nerves out of action and leading to weakness of the muscles they should supply.

It will be seen how confusion can arise, complicated sometimes by the use of the word 'nervous' in ordinary speech to imply shakiness or apprehension. Fortunately the progress in treatment of mental illnesses, and the knowledge that these are illnesses just as are bronchitis or lumbago, is allowing much freer discussion of the situations as they arise, and the need to dissemble when describing mental illness should soon pass.

Nettle Rash (Urticaria, 'Hives'). An itching condition of the skin sometimes resulting from contact, internal or external, with something to which the patient is *allergic*. This may be a food, such as shellfish or strawberries, a pollen inhaled, or a plant touched, a bee sting, or an antibiotic such as penicillin. The rash takes the form of raised red weals with white centres, and can happen on any part of the body. Scratching the skin produces more weals whose shape follows that of the scratch marks. In severe cases, the lips and tongue may swell sufficiently to hinder breathing, and it then becomes urgent to get the patient to hospital or doctor. (See also under *Stings*.)

A patient will usually know what allergy is responsible, and be able to avoid it. (Anyone who has proved allergic to penicillin should never be given another dose unless he has been desensitized, and should always warn his doctor of his allergy.) In many cases the cause cannot be recognized, and it is thought that nervous stress may be responsible.

The treatment of an attack is with antihistamine preparations, and anyone prone to attacks will already have these from his doctor. Lacking them, dabbing the rash with calamine lotion or cold tea will help. In severe attacks, and always if lips or tongue are affected, the doctor is needed urgently (**S** to **UU**, depending on severity).

Neuralgia. Pain felt in a part of the body in which there is no obvious cause for pain, and presumed to arise from some disorder of the nerve which conveys sensation from that part of the body to the brain. Thus, pain in the jaw caused by an inflamed tooth is not neuralgia — the nerve is doing its job of carrying information to the brain. The same pain in the absence of any dental disease is neuralgia — the nerve is transmitting false information, due to some (not yet understood) disorder of its mechanism.

Home treatment of neuralgia is that of the pain it causes — *aspirin* or *paracetamol*. Only the doctor or dentist can tell whether the pain is caused by neuralgia or something else (C). (See also *Herpes zoster*.)

Neurosis. Name of a group of mental disorders which are not necessarily severe, and are not regarded as implying insanity. They are mentioned here, not because they are suitable for home treatment — a doctor should always be consulted — but because recovery is assisted if patient and those around him are aware of the nature of the illness.

There are three main types:

1 **Anxiety neurosis** ('anxiety state'), in which the natural sensation of anxiety is prolonged and distorted, giving rise to foreboding, loss of confidence, and bodily symptoms such as trembling, palpitation, and sweating.
2 **Reactive depression,** in which the symptoms of *depression* are produced by outside stresses, rather than by internal disorder of the mind.
3 **Hysterical neurosis,** resulting in symptoms (pain, loss of use of a part of the body, etc) for which there is no organic cause. (See *Hysteria*.)

All these are produced by a load of stress greater than the particular constitution is designed to bear. The level at which accumulated stress will produce neurosis varies in any individual according to his state of resistance — for instance it will be low after illness, and high after the achievement of a difficult task.

The three zones of daily experience in which the presence of stress is most likely to be effective are: work, family, and sex life. Stress is most likely to arise from frustration, or from a conflict between what the patient would like to do and what he believes to be the right course of behaviour.

See also *Anxiety, Depression, Palpitation, Contemplation, 'Nerves'*.

Night Rising. A few people have a life-long need to pass urine once during the night. For them, it is a constitutional necessity. Most people do not; when they go to bed their kidneys produce a smaller volume of urine than during the day, and their bladders are able to contain this volume until morning, without signalling that they need to be emptied. If such a person suddenly finds the need to rise one or more times each night, it may be due to irritation of the bladder, as by *cystitis* or enlargement of the *prostate gland*, weakening of the muscles which regulate the bladder (commoner in women), or reduced power of the kidneys, which are then unable to produce sufficient urine during the day, and have to continue output at the day rate for part of the night. Clearly, a case for investigation in various ways, and the doctor should be consulted (**C**), taking a *specimen of urine*.

Night Sweats. Anyone may wake in a sweat if the night is unseasonably hot, if he has eaten or drunk too much, or if he develops a feverish cold or 'flu'. If one persistently does so over a period of days or weeks, it may be due to feverishness at night, and this *can* be the result of a chronic infection, such as pulmonary tuberculosis, so the complaint calls for investigation (**C**).

Normal Saline. This term is now obsolete as it has different meanings in Pharmacy and Scientific Chemistry. (See *Isotonic Saline*.)

Nosebleed. Most nosebleeds are from the blood vessels on the septum ('party wall' between the nostrils), and many from the front of it. Nosebleeds in younger people are not usually serious; some adolescents have a nosebleed two or three times a year. In older people, blood vessels are brittle and circulation pressure may be higher, so that they bleed for longer, and may lose more.

Most nosebleeds will stop in the course of half an hour or so, whatever one does. Unfortunately, one cannot forecast which ones will not, so the same treatment should be adopted for all:

1 Sit the patient comfortably at a table with a cushion for his

elbows, leaning forwards. Tilt his face a little downwards.
2 In this position, the blood should run out of the nostrils, and not down his throat. He holds a saucer against his upper lip to catch it.
3 It will now be apparent from which nostril the blood is coming. Apply pressure on the soft side of the nose, closing the nostril against the 'party wall', and this should stop the bleeding. Keep the pressure up for five to seven minutes, then gently release. If the bleeding restarts, repeat the pressure. While this is going on, a *cold pack* is placed on the back of the patient's neck, and he is told to breathe through his mouth below the saucer and to try to swallow as seldom as possible — each time he swallows, he causes suction at the back of his nose, and increases the bleeding. (Holding a cork between the teeth helps.)
4 The blood from the saucer is saved in a jam jar or pint measure, so that the total loss can be estimated. Don't let the patient fuss about with old sheets, sponges, etc.
5 Failure of pressure to control the bleeding after about half an hour indicates that the doctor should be informed, stating how long the bleeding has continued, and how much blood loss has been measured.
6 Meanwhile, the cold pack is repeated, renewing the cold water every five minutes, and a trial is made with a *hydrogen peroxide* plug.
7 If at any time in the course of a nosebleed the lost blood measures over half a pint, or the patient becomes faint, the doctor should be informed. For faintness, the head will have to be lowered, and the patient turned to the semi-prone position (see *Unconsciousness*) to prevent blood being inhaled. Bleeding will probably start again, and must be controlled as described at the beginning of para (3) until the doctor arrives (**U** or **UU**).
8 Once the bleeding has stopped, *and it nearly always does*, the patient should remain sitting upright with head and back supported, for two or three hours. That night, he should be well propped up with pillows in bed.

Nursing. A patient who has to keep to his bed for more than a week or 10 days requires the help of a professional nurse, and if a trained relative or friend is not available, one can employ a private nurse or ask for calls by the district nurse, through one's doctor.

For a short stay in bed, the objectives are cleanliness, care of the skin and prevention of immobility. The body should be washed all over each day with hot water and soap, keeping separate cloths for face and body. The genital and anal areas are best washed with disposable material, such as lint or cellulose wadding. Facility should be provided for cleansing hands after excretion, and teeth or dentures cleaned at least night and morning. After washing, the skin of back, buttocks, thighs, and heels is rubbed gently with surgical spirit or such cream as the doctor may order, the latter always being used for any reddened areas. Any blistering or breaking of the skin should be reported to the doctor (V). Pressure of heels on mattress is reduced by making the foot of the bed loosely. The lower sheet should be kept as free from wrinkles as possible, and should be changed every third or fourth day. Only use a waterproof under-sheet if there is soiling. It should be combined with the use of a draw-sheet across the middle third of the bed, which can be pulled on the roller towel principle, allowing a fresh area of sheet to be exposed several times a day. If this is not done, the skin becomes too moist and is easily damaged. (In many areas the District Nursing Service can supply disposable under-sheet pads, and these can be used in combination with 'one way' draw-sheets, bought from the chemist.)

Usually, young and middle-aged patients are sufficiently mobile in bed to prevent pressure damage to the skin. From the start, they should be encouraged to clench calf and thigh muscles from time to time, and move ankles and legs, preventing sluggishness in the circulation of the leg veins. In older people, one should try to ensure that they change position from side to back and to the other side, every hour, to lessen the risk of breakdown of the skin into pressure (bed) sores.

A bell and any tablets ordered for emergency use are left within easy reach. All other tablets are stored well away and their doses issued as required. It is not *necessary* to have a daily bowel action, but most people feel more comfortable if they do so. Lack of exercise and reduced food intake may combine with feverishness to reduce bowel activity, and it is reasonable to give one or two doses of *paraffin* emulsion (one to three 5 ml spoonfuls) each day, or one or two Senokot tablets each night, adjusting the dose by results.

If the doctor advises that the patient may sit out of bed for the purpose, excretion is best dealt with on a bedside commode; if not, by urinal and bed pans. Some people at first feel hesitant in being able to use them, and may need to be left alone with the assurance that they will not be interrupted.

Obesity (overweight). 'Obesity is always due to eating too much.'

This saying by a teaching physician represents a widely held opinion. Not 'too much' in a gluttonous sense, but more than the body can use as fuel in the course of the day's work, so that a surplus is converted to fat and laid down as a reserve. Although this provides a useful working idea, there are zones of uncertainty as to the part played by water retention in susceptible people, and there are certain factors, not understood, which can make obesity less easy to master; such as a constitutional tendency to store unused food as fat, rather than burn it away, effects of abdominal operation, following childbirth, etc.

There now seems no doubt that overweight people have a seriously higher rate of coronary heart disease, high blood pressure and some other complaints.

Disorders of the internal glands and brain damage produce a more complicated situation, which is usually not simple obesity.

A healthy person who is moderately overweight can reasonably try the effect of a low carbohydrate diet, reducing or omitting sugar (use saccharine for sweetening), bread, potatoes, cakes, pastries; and stop eating between meals. This should give a loss of several pounds in the first few weeks. If it does not, the doctor may be consulted. A severe reducing diet should never be followed except under medical advice.

Appetite is nature's way of ensuring that we take steps to find and eat food. In the competitive conditions in which homo sapiens developed, the risk of over-eating was as small as it is in India today. In some conditions of nervous stress, the appetite is increased, food acting as a comforter. This may be very marked if the patient has recently deprived himself of the comfort of tobacco, and the wives of lapsed smokers complain bitterly of the effect on their housekeeping budgets. It is a fact, however, that after a few weeks of abstinence the appetite contracts, and it becomes much easier to keep to the reduced intake.

Exercise Roughly, an hour's hard work is needed to use up two slices of bread, so hopes of reducing weight substantially by exercise, without modifying the diet which has been at fault, are usually not realized. *The best exercise for reducing weight is to turn the head slowly from side to side when offered second helpings.*

Overweight (that is, overfed or wrongly fed) babies are handicapped babies. Their resistance to illness is lessened, and they may be starting on a life-long habit of obesity and over-eating.

Overweight (see *Obesity*).

Pain. The purpose of pain is to draw attention to something wrong. The body is unfortunately better at doing this than removing the cause, but it is not always consistent, and some serious conditions are quite painless in their early stages (see. *Lump*).

Here is a brief survey of the more frequent causes of pain. Pain due to *injuries* is covered separately under that heading.

Head. Many causes, of which the most frequent by far is ordinary headache, usually produced by worry, tension, fatigue, or frustration. It can be relieved by *aspirin* or *paracetamol*. Its big brother *migraine* needs special treatment.

Headache is a feature of *fever* and of *meningism*.

Headache felt in both front and back of the head may be due to *spondylosis*, a rheumatic situation involving the small joints at the upper end of the neck. It will often respond to the above treatment, as for headache, combined with the use of a single *butterfly pillow*. Frequent attacks may need physiotherapy or other treatment. A less frequent cause of pain in the back of the head is raised blood pressure, whose diagnosis and treatment are medical matters (**C** or **D**).

The central forehead pain of *sinusitis* may complicate a cold or hay fever, or may come on without warning. It is usually worse in the morning and on hanging the head down. Severe cases need medical help (**S** or occasionally **D**). Milder ones will respond to *steam inhalations* three or four times daily for five to ten minutes each time. After each inhalation the patient lies on a bed or couch with the head thrown back over the edge, so that it is upside down. In this position, six to ten drops of ephedrine nasal drops are run into each nostril, and the position held for five minutes. On sitting up slowly, some of the drops will run forwards out of the nose, the remainder backwards and can be swallowed. This routine should not be continued for more than three days without advice.

Neck (see *Spondylosis*).

Shoulders. Rheumatism apart, spondylosis of the lower neck can give rise to shoulder pain, more severe if one of the intervertebral discs has become softened and misshaped. Capsulitis of the shoulder or 'frozen shoulder' seems to be a complication of this, though the connexion is not understood. In this, the movements of the upper arm and the shoulder joint are limited by pain and muscle spasm. While waiting for medical advice (**C**), avoid heavy lifting and repeated movements as in sweeping, etc, the use of a *butterfly pillow* and of *aspirin* or *paracetamol* will relieve. Frozen shoulder is helped by taking the weight of the upper arm in a sling for several hours each day.

Armpit. Associated with one or more tender swellings:
1. Inflamed lymph gland.
2. Boil.
3. Hidradenitis, numerous small red tender swellings from infection of the glands in the skin, some coming to a head.

For all these, (**S**) for consideration of antibiotic treatment. Meanwhile, *hot* isotonic saline *packs*. It should be remembered that the female breast extends into the armpit, and pain can be caused after childbirth either by congestion of the breast (relieved by *hot packs,* and gently expressing the milk) or breast infection, when a patch of skin is red, hot, and tender, the underlying tissue hard and the temperature raised (**S** or **D**) Meanwhile, frequent *hot packs* and continue to use the breast for feeding.

Elbow. Tennis elbow — an inflammation of the group of muscles attached to the outer knob of the elbow. It can last many months before clearing up on its own, and medical advice should be sought (**C**). Sometimes steroid injections help to clear it.

Forearm. Pain in moving the wrist, coming on after repeated twisting or flexing movements of the hand, as when driving screws or singling root vegetables, often accompanied by a creaking sound in the muscles, is due to inflammation of the tendon sheaths (**S**).

Hand. Aching and tingling in the wrist and palm, extending to the fingers and elbow, can be caused by pressure on a nerve as it passes through the wrist ('carpal tunnel syndrome'). It is often worse after a night in bed, easing during the day. It may need relief by a minor operation if medical measures fail (**C**). Similar pain can arise from spondylosis.

Fingers. Throbbing pain in the soft flesh, worse on hanging the hand, and tender on pressure, is usually due to 'poisoned finger' (see *Finger, poisoned*) (**S**).

Chest. The chest is a cage of ribs and muscles containing the heart and lungs. It expands and contracts with every breath, and pain which is worse on breathing or only happens with a breath, is often due to rheumatism in the muscles or rib hinges, or to inflammation of the smooth lining, causing friction against the lungs ('pleurisy'). This sort of pain varies from mild inconvenience to complete incapacity, and needs medical diagnosis. The mild cases can usually visit the doctor (**S**), unless there is fever or constitutional upset. The more severe need a visit the same day (**D**). Meanwhile, *aspirin* or *paracetamol* internally, and *kaolin poultice* or *hot pack* to the site of pain. A raw pain on breathing, felt behind the breast bone, is usual in tracheitis (see *Cough*). Continuous pain behind the breast bone, often severe, and sometimes extending towards the jaw, shoulder and arm, or down to the upper abdomen, can be due to a *coronary attack*, or sometimes to troubles with one of the spinal 'discs' (see *Spondylosis*). As diagnosis may be difficult, the patient should be supported in a comfortable position until the doctor can see him (**UU** to **D**, according to severity).

Pain under the lower edge of the right-hand ribs can be due to gall-stones or inflamed gall-bladder. The pain is sometimes felt also in the right shoulder. The doctor is needed (**U** to **D**, according to severity). Meanwhile, a guarded *hot water bottle* to the part, and occasional small sips of spirit. Chest pain in the zone covering two or three ribs on one side may last for several days just before an attack of shingles (see *Herpes zoster*). If mild, it is justifiable to treat with *aspirin* or *paracetamol* for a few days while watching for the rash to appear. If severe, the pain will need medical help in its own right (**S**).

Breast. In addition to conditions noted under *breast*, and in *armpit* above, general painful tension with or without swelling is experienced by some women in the 10 days before *menstruation*. It is due to increase of fluid in the tissues and can often be prevented by medical treatment (**C**). A similar feeling is noticed in the early weeks of pregnancy, and later the increasing weight of the breasts can make them painful. This will be helped by wearing a *supportive* brassiere, made to hold up the breasts from below, and to allow plenty of room for the nipples.

Abdomen. The home treatment of abdominal (belly) pain is so difficult that with the exception of *gastroenteritis* and mild enteritis, the attempt should not be made. Except in these conditions, if abdominal pain, continuous or intermittent, lasts for more than two hours, the doctor should be informed, giving details. In a case where something such as a gastric ulcer has burst, the patient's response to the suggestion of waiting that long will be a sufficient indication that help is needed much more quickly. There is usually a sudden onset of very severe abdominal pain, increasing, sometimes with pain on breathing, or extending to one or other shoulder, and an attempt to feel the abdomen shows that the muscles covering it are iron hard (**UU**). While waiting for the doctor, apply guarded *hot water bottle* to the site of pain and to the soles of the patient's feet. He will usually be most comfortable propped up in bed (see *Backrest*), and should be given nothing by mouth. (See also *labour* contractions.) Never give an aperient to anyone with abdominal pain.

On passing water, or just after it, often felt as 'scalding', and associated with a frequent urge to pass small quantities, is usually due to inflammation of the bladder (*Cystitis*). A *specimen of urine* should be taken to the doctor (**S**). Meanwhile, a good intake of water or fruit drinks, and a level teaspoonful of bicarbonate of soda taken three times in the day (but not continued for more than one day) will ease the symptoms. (The urine may at first be bloodstained.)

On passing a motion, often due to *piles* or to a fissure (crack) in the anal opening, itself a complication of piles. Needs medical advice (**C**). Meanwhile keep motions soft with liquid *paraffin*. Insert a compound bismuth subgallate suppository ('Anusol') immediately on waking, and again as soon as the bowel has acted. Pain is eased by a *hot pack* to the anus and by taking *aspirin* or *paracetamol*.

Testicles. See under that heading.

Legs and **Feet.** Most of the causes are described under separate headings.

Pain in any of the joints can be caused by *arthritis*, and by *gout*, particularly in the great toe joint, which can be the site of a *bunion*.

Pain in the *knee* is covered under that title.

Pain in the back of the buttock, thigh, and leg can be caused by *sciatica, cramp,* and *thrombosis*, also be a torn calf muscle. The latter arises suddenly when a springing movement is made, often when playing a game or jumping. It feels as if the back of the calk had been struck, and the immediate pain is relieved by *cold packs*, but a doctor's advice is usually needed (**S** or **V**). It is important not to mistake *thrombosis* of a vein in the calf for *cramp* or *sciatica*, and the entry on *thrombosis* should be read.

Pain over the shin can be due to *motorist's leg*, and throbbing pain combined with fever, and occasionally some reddening of the skin, may be a sign of bone infection (osteomyelitis) in children (**D**). An *ulcer* of the lower leg is often due to *varicose* *veins* (**C**). Pain in one or both calves which starts after walking a certain distance, goes off on resting and returns after further walking, is intermittent claudication, due to slowing of the circulation. It is commonest in the elderly, due to atheroma ('furring up') of the arteries, but in younger people is sometimes caused by a short length of localized obstruction (**S**).

Herpes zoster (Shingles) can cause pain anywhere, unexplained until a rash appears some days later.

Flat foot is a common cause of pain, as are *corns, warts* (verruca), and ingrowing toenails (see *Nails*).

Pain in the foot of a *diabetic* or elderly patient calls for medical attention, as it may indicate that the circulation is failing, with a danger of gangrene. Part of the foot, or one or more toes, may be either much paler or much darker than the remainder, and the pain can be very severe (**D** or **U**, depending on severity). Meanwhile, *aspirin* or *paracetamol*; the foot to be kept warm with blankets, but no additional heat given.

Palpitation. A loose term which can cover a number of disorders, few of which are serious. A patient more often complains of palpitation than a doctor diagnoses it, and it usually means an increased awareness of the beating of the lower left corner of the heart, the point at which it is nearest the ribs, and where its beat can usually be seen and felt. As such, the commonest cause is *anxiety* and nervous tension, and attention should be given to relief of these if the doctor's investigations show no sign of heart mischief. A short period set aside daily for *contemplation*; consideration of the day's expected difficulties, with decision as to which of them it is in one's own power to alter; the preparation of a list (written for preference) of what has to be done the next day; will all yield a benefit in tranquillity which will help overcome the effects of stress.

Paroxysmal tachycardia is a rare condition in which the rate at which the heart beats suddenly increases from the usual 70–80 per minute to between 150 and 250 per minute. The patient may know that he has a tendency to these attacks, which do not usually indicate heart disease, and may know of the tricks which can be used to stop them. These include bending over, pressing on the eyeballs through the closed eyelids (to be avoided in the severely short-sighted, as it might then injure the eyes), breathing out strongly against a closed throat (as if forcing a constipated bowel action), and tickling the back of the throat with a finger to provoke retching. A patient for whom these do not provide relief may become distressed, and should be rested in a sitting position until the doctor can see him (U or D). If he becomes faint he should be put in the semi-prone position (see p. 247).

Paracetamol Tablets, 500 mg. A useful substitute for *aspirin* for relief of pain. They are less likely to cause stomach inflammation and can usually be taken by 'ulcer' or 'gastric' patients. 1 or 2 may be taken at intervals of 4 to 6 hours, with a maximum of 8 in 24 hours. They should only be used for long-term treatment on medical advice.

In liquid form for children it can be given as 'paracetamol elixir paediatric, BPC'. The dose for children from 6 months to 1 year, is one 5 ml spoonful; from 1 to 5 years two 5 ml spoonfuls, not more than three doses in 24 hours. It should not be kept for more than a few weeks.

Paraffin, Medicinal or Liquid. A syrupy oil, nothing to do with kerosene. Useful as an occasional laxative for softening hard motions, taken either as liquid paraffin, one or two 5 ml spoonfuls three times a day, or as paraffin emulsion, which some find pleasanter, two or three 5 ml spoonfuls three times a day.

After long-continued use, paraffin has occasionally given rise to internal trouble. (See also *constipation* and *aperient*.)

Also used for cleansing the skin in cases of *eczema* or dermatitis, when soap and water cannot be used.

Paralysis. The old name of palsy is still sometimes heard. A situation in which a muscle or group of muscles cannot be used because the nerve which should take instructions to it from the brain, or the relevant part of the brain itself, is damaged.

Peptic Ulcer. This term covers both *duodenal* and *gastric ulcers*, which are separately described.

Diagnosis (C) is usually confirmed by 'barium meal' X-ray, in which a feed mixed with radio-opaque barium is viewed on an X-ray screen as it passes through the digestive organs. *Warning:* some people find themselves appallingly constipated by the barium. Take 10 ml of *paraffin* emulsion three times each day after the X-ray until it has all passed through.

Treatment of peptic ulcer is either medical or surgical. Some cases are as obviously medical as others are surgical, but many fall between, and the decision calls for keen judgement of the total situation: patient, disease, way of life, stresses, etc. Whatever treatment is given, ask fully about any future limitations of diet or activity, and cooperate in them.

Smoking, worry, alcohol, and aspirin are all bad for peptic ulcers.

Pets (see *Animals, domestic*).

Phlebitis. Inflammation in a vein, sometimes leading to formation of a blood clot. See under *Thrombosis* for important precautions.

Phlegm (sputum). Matter which is coughed up. In ordinary health, the lining of the nose and bronchial tubes is freed from dust and germs by a moving carpet of sticky mucus. This is constantly formed and passes upward from the bronchial tubes and backwards from the nose to the throat, where it is swallowed and sterilized by the digestive juices in the stomach. In some people, rather more of this mucus is formed than they welcome and they become very worried at having to swallow it, calling it 'catarrh' and fearing that it is some sort of disease. It should be regarded as a harmless — indeed necessary — mechanism which in their case is working to excess. If they can reassure themselves, they will forget about it for long periods. Drastic steps at self-treatment can be harmful.

If the inhaled germs are too strong to be dealt with by the moving mucus, they will establish themselves in the windpipe ('tracheitis', the ordinary cough following a cold), or bronchial tubes (bronchitis), or lungs themselves (broncho-pneumonia). In these situations, much more mucus will be formed, mixed with dead germs and the white corpuscles which have hurried to kill the germs, so that the sputum becomes creamy, yellow, or green, and has to be coughed up to clear the air passages. (See also *Cough*). Blood in the phlegm — see *Bleeding*.

Piles (see *Haemorrhoids*).

Pink Eye. A common form of conjunctivitis, very infectious. See *Eye*. The towels, facecloth, pillowslip, etc, of the patient should be boiled each day until the condition is cured, to reduce the risk of infection or re-infection (**S—** with care!).

Plastic Bags. Containers of polythene or similar film in which foodstuffs are packed. If children put their heads in these, they may be suffocated, and several have been. If the bags are thrown away in the countryside, they may be eaten by animals and cause them internal injury, or even death.

Pleurisy (see *Pain in chest*).

Pneumonia (see *Cough*).

Poisoning. The taking of poison by mouth may be accidental or suicidal; rarely homicidal. Accidental poisoning occurs from a wider range of substances than suicidal, which is commonly from *aspirin*, 'sedative' or 'nerve' tablets, sleeping tablets or capsules.

When found, the patient will be either conscious or unconscious. If the latter, and breathing well, the priority is to arrange transport to hospital, or failing that to call a doctor (**UU**). While waiting, maintain body heat with blankets, but no hot water bottles. Vomiting in a semi-conscious patient can cause suffocation, and if it threatens, the patient is rolled over so that the mouth faces downwards and to the side. If breathing fails, *artificial respiration* is required urgently and is continued until help arrives.

Immediate treatment of a conscious poisoned patient depends on the extent of his co-operation, the nature of the poison, and the amount of help available. If the first and last are satisfactory, *and provided poisoning is not by paraffin, white spirit or other petroleum product nor a corrosive acid or alkali* (acid or caustic burns may show on face and mouth), an attempt is made to cause vomiting. Advice on how to do this has undergone one of its periodical alterations. An adult or older child will usually vomit if the back of the throat is tickled with a feather or finger — preferably his own. There is a special draught for children — Ipecacuanha emetic draught, paediatric, BPC 1973 (see First Aid list), but it is now advised that its use should be supervised by a doctor if one can reach the patient within, say, forty minutes. If delay is expected, make urgent arrangements for transport to hospital, and while awaiting this, give 10 ml of the draught for a child aged 6–18 months, 15 ml for an old child, followed if possible by 100 ml (4 oz) of water. Do make sure that vomiting takes place with the body tilted down towards the head, and the face and mouth turned downwards. Keep the vomit in a clean vessel for analysis.

Salt and water should not be used to provoke vomiting, as it can make matters worse, and has even proved fatal.

If rapid transport to a nearby hospital or Poison Treatment Centre is available, nothing more than these quick measures should be attempted. If there is a delay, proceed as follows, where appropriate:

If it is known that acid — usually spirits of salts, or vitriol — has been taken, give a raw egg into which the finely crushed shell has been beaten, or milk, not more than ten ounces (for an adult) during the first half hour. Do not give chalk or bicarbonate of soda.

If the poison is known to be alkali — such as caustic soda — give four ounces of vinegar, or two to three ounces of lemon juice in sips, slowly. If there is a smell of carbolic, it is reasonable to cause vomiting, preferably mechanically, but milk should *not* be given.

A written note telling what has been done, should be sent with the patient to hospital, together with the vomit container, and any remaining posion for identification. (See also *Gas or Fume Poisoning* and *Food Poisoning*.)

Poliomyelitis (Infantile Paralysis). A virus infection which can damage or destroy the nerve connexions between brain and muscle, resulting in *paralysis* of the muscles concerned. At times when the disease is prevalent, many people harbour the virus in throat or bowel without being affected by it. Infection is by airborne droplets, or contamination of food and water by faulty sanitary habits or defective sanitation. The majority of cases are non-paralytic and may not be recognized as poliomyelitis at all.

The patient has a sore throat, lassitude, head- and backache, often with *meningism*. These may last up to a week before subsiding spontaneously. If the case is a paralytic one, weakness and pain in one or more limbs, and sometimes of chest and other muscles, usually start after about 4 days, though the interval is variable and occasionally absent.

A patient who complains of headache, has a raised temperature and whose back hurts when he nods his chin on to his chest, has *meningism*. Most will be due to a comparatively harmless infection, a few to 'polio' and a few to meningitis.

1. Ask doctor to call the same day (**D**).
2. Patient to *rest in bed*. Neglect of this can greatly increase the paralysis should the illness prove to be poliomyelitis.
3. Treat head- and back-ache with *aspirin* or *paracetamol* tablets, and *cold compress* to brow and temples.

See also *Vaccination*, about active immunization and avoidance of some other injections if poliomyelitis is prevalent.

Posture. Posture in general is covered under *Relaxation* (2).

Effect of posture on the working of the brain: practitioners of yoga hold that posture plays a part, together with control of breathing and muscles, in directing the circulation to the best advantage of the brain. Though it is not possible to parallel all the yogic theory with the present state of scientific knowledge, many people believe that they concentrate best in a certain position, eg, as when sitting at a desk; and anyone accustomed to pray kneeling finds it difficult to do so standing. Some of this is a matter of habit, but it may reasonably be expected that one's power of decision, at any rate, will be better if one is in a posture which does not reduce the prospect of physical action; anyone surprised in bed with the need to take a critical decision will not wish to do so until he has put his feet on the ground. Those who believe they work or think best in a particular posture should adopt it whenever possible — why make life more difficult?

Pregnancy. The first indication of a pregnancy is usually the absence of *menstruation*. In the first few weeks, the breasts may be unusually sensitive, but this happens to many women before the onset of menstruation, so that a delayed period can cause uncertainty. A doctor can usually tell whether a pregnancy is or is not present by making an internal examination 10 or 11 weeks after the start of the last period. Before that, a laboratory test on the urine gives an accurate answer in a high proportion of cases, though an occasional false reading is possible. These tests are usually available on medical grounds through the hospital service; if needed for social reasons, they can be made for a fee by a private laboratory.

Once a pregnancy is diagnosed, the mother will come under the care of her doctor, midwife, or hospital maternity department for regular supervision and advice.

The *average* duration of a pregnancy is 40 weeks from the date of the last normal menstruation. The usual calculation is to subtract 3 calendar months from this date, then add a week, to give the *approximate* date of confinement. The sensitivity of the breasts in the early weeks has already been mentioned, and care of the breasts should start early. A brassiere giving firm support from below, and no pressure from in front, should be worn. After daily washing with soap and hot water, the nipples should be gently pulled outwards for a few minutes. The doctor's advice should be sought if the nipple is 'retracted' or sunk in the breast. From the sixth month onward, daily care of the breasts should include 'expressing'.

The breast is grasped in both hands and gently squeezed towards the nipple, from which a little fluid will often then flow.

The two principles of maternity wear are to support the breasts and abdomen from below with a suitable brassiere and maternity belt; and to hang all the other clothes from the shoulders, leaving the waist free.

'Morning sickness' is a traditional feature of the first three months, but is less common than formerly, partly because the apprehensions which contributed to it have been dispelled by free discussion. If it is troublesome, it nearly always responds to medical treatment (C). The ideal diet in pregnancy is a well mixed one, with plenty of fresh food, enough vitamins, and at least a pint of milk daily, in drinks or other ways. The carbohydrate foods, bread, potatoes, cakes, sugar, sweets, etc, are the least useful and should be taken in moderation. Extra iron is often needed, and is ordered by the doctor.

Provided there is no tendency to *miscarriage*, normal non-violent activity should be continued, short of producing exhaustion. Extreme physical exertion is best avoided, as the stretching of muscles and ligaments which occurs has made them rather less effective than usual in controlling the body's movements.

Sexual intercourse can continue up to six weeks before confinement is expected, avoiding the times at which menstruation would have occurred. If there is a tendency to miscarriage, it should be avoided throughout the pregnancy, unless advised otherwise. Following confinement, three or four weeks should be allowed before resumption. If discomfort is caused, wait another week or two. Seek medical advice if it persists.

In the later months, every effort should be made to arrange matters so that an afternoon rest can be taken with the feet up. There is a natural tendency for the feet and legs to become heavy, even a little swollen by night. If this happens suddenly, or is more than mild, the doctor should be consulted (S, taking *specimen of urine*; UU if accompanied by severe headache, vaginal bleeding, or abdominal pain).

Although the great majority of pregnancies are passed

naturally and uneventfully, it is as well to be aware of some of the things which can occasionally go wrong:

1. Bleeding from the vagina always calls for medical advice. Lie down and send word to the doctor, saying whether you are losing less than, as much as, or more than a normal 'period' and whether there is any pain. This will help him to decide how urgent the matter is.
2. Pain on passing water, usually due to *cystitis* or pyelitis (see *kidney disease*). (**D** or **S** according to severity. Keep a specimen of urine for examination.)
3. Sudden flow of water from the vagina, in later pregnancy. If booked for home confinement, lie down and notify midwife or doctor. If booked for hospital, summon transport and get in as soon as possible, as labour sometimes starts rapidly after this occurrence.

Relaxation during pregnancy. This is now taught by many doctors and obstetricians, usually at the same time as prenatal exercises. Anyone wishing to practise on her own should follow the scheme outlined in *Relaxation* (1), or in *Easier Childbirth* by Elliot Phillip and Ruth Forbes — Family Doctor booklet. The object of practising relaxation during pregnancy is to prevent interference during labour by one of nature's primitive safeguards, no longer required in conditions of civilized life. At the end of pregnancy, the womb may be represented as an inverted bag made of long strips of muscle, arranged like the staves of a barrel, and closed at its lower end by a circular muscle which acts as a purse-string. At the onset of *labour*, messages come down nerves from the brain, telling the long muscle strips to start shortening to open the purse-string, and then to expel the baby, who is lying head-down in the womb. A mother starting labour is clearly not going to be very mobile for some hours, and under primitive conditions there was an advantage in a mechanism whereby on the appearance of a sabre-toothed tiger from the jungle she could close down the proceedings and ascend a convenient tree. This was achieved by a second set of nerves running from the brain to the circular muscle, activation of which would close the womb and stop the labour proceeding. This alarm mechanism is set off by worry or anxiety, and can then lead to delay in the progress of labour and strain the muscles of the womb, so that contractions which need only have been uncomfortable become painful. It has been found that the action of the alarm system can be prevented by the regular practice of relaxation and breath control before and during labour, and by other aids to tranquillity, such as a clear explanation of the mechanism of labour to the mother.

The thalidomide tragedy will have made most people aware that *drugs, including tobacco, and tablets should not be taken during the first three months of a pregnancy, except under medical guidance*, and opinion is now in favour of extending this caution to the whole pregnancy.

Each year, a small number of babies are born with congenital defects, due to infection of the mother during pregnancy with toxoplasmosis. The fact that this disease can be caught from cats who catch and eat rodents suggests that contact with cats should be minimal.

As knowledge about recognition and treatment of babies at risk of slow development and backwardness has increased, it has become more important to date the start of a pregnancy accurately. Every woman should keep a diary note of the first day of each period throughout the child-bearing phase of her life. (See *Home Confinements*, p. 25.)

Further Reading
You and your pregnancy month by month by Elliott Phillip, FRCOG, and Ruth Forbes, Family Doctor Booklet.

Proflavine Cream. A useful first aid cream for application to abrasions and cuts, as it retains its antiseptic properties in contact with the fluids exuded from raw areas. It is best applied on a pad of surgical gauze. If it is feared that the dressing may stick to the wound, a layer of paraffin gauze may

- **If a patient is not within the scope of home care, or worsens in spite of it, or if there is any uncertainty, a doctor should be consulted.**

be placed directly on the wound, then the proflavine cream dressing. It is better to bandage the dressing than use adhesive plaster, anyway for the first few days, as this reduces the accumulation of fluid in the damaged area. (See also *Dressings*.)

Prolapse. In everyday speech, refers to prolapse of the womb (uterus), which is held in place by a system of muscles and ligaments. If these slacken, usually from childbirth or the effects of age, the uterus slides downwards into, and may protrude from, the vagina. The situation can also involve the bladder and rectum, and may lead to difficulty in controlling excretion.

The type of operation needed to repair prolapse varies with the nature and extent of the damage. The interval before physical work and sexual intercourse can be resumed is equally variable, and advice on this should be taken from the consultant or ward sister (as mentioned under *Hysterectomy*) before leaving hospital.

Prostate Gland. In men, a roughly spherical gland lying immediately below the urinary bladder and encircling the bladder outlet tube (urethra) like a collar. After middle age the prostate often increases in size, and may cause irritation of the bladder, with frequent and incomplete emptying. It may also at this time press on the urethra so that the bladder cannot be emptied, resulting in 'retention'. This is most likely to happen in conditions of cold and fatigue, particularly when an unusual quantity of fluid has been taken. The returning reveller on a winter's night who has forgotten to empty his bladder before the journey home is a typical candidate. If the situation arises before he reaches home, he should go to the casualty department of the nearest hospital. If at home, he should immerse himself in a deep, comfortably hot bath with his head resting on his sponge, loofah, or pillow, relax completely, and try to let (not force) the bladder empty into the hot water. If after half an hour he is not successful his doctor should be asked to call, the message stating without disguise what the situation is, as the doctor may wish to prepare equipment.

In some areas where hospital facilities allow, cases of retention are admitted to hospital for immediate operation, just as appendicitis would be. Otherwise, the doctor will relieve the retention by passing a small tube up the penis into the bladder — not usually painful — and arrangements are made later for the necessary investigation and treatment. Older men who may remember tales of the horrors and risks of the prostate operation may be comforted to know that nowadays this is no worse than any other abdominal operation, and gives a high proportion of very good results. In general, the operation ('prostatectomy') does not alter sexual capacity, but it involves the trying of the sperm tubes, so that the patient is thereafter sterile.

Prostatic enlargement may produce urges to sexual behaviour inconsistent with that expected of one of mature years. If these threaten to escape control, one's doctor should be consulted without hesitation (C).

Psoriasis ('*sore-eye-as-iss*'). A constitutional skin disorder, the tendency to which is sometimes inherited. *It is not infectious.* In mild cases, there are patches of silvery flakes on the elbows and knees. These can develop on any part of the skin, including the scalp, during bad stages of the complaint; and such are most likely when the patient is worried or under strain. No permanent cure is yet known, but there is a variety of treatments available to control the disease, and medical advice should be sought (C). The possessor of a tranquil mind is seldom much troubled by psoriasis. Sufferers should consider joining the Psoriasis Association (p. 265).

Puberty. The onset of sexual development in a child at an age varying from 11 to 14 years. A girl's breasts develop, pubic hair grows, she starts to menstruate, and her body begins to conform to the shape of an adult. A boy's genital organs increase in size, pubic hair grows, and the increasing size of his voice box (Adam's apple) will lead to his voice 'breaking' to a lower pitch. Boys quite often develop swollen and tender nipples (one or both) for a time. It is a natural occurrence in almost all cases, though it is as well to consult the doctor, who will be able to spot the occasional case needing observation. (See also *Menstruation*, and the chapter *From the Second Year to Adolescence*.)

Pulse. 'Taking the pulse' tells how fast the heart is beating, if it is beating. The rate normally lies within the range of 60 to 90 per minute. The traditional place for pulse taking is at the wrist, an inch above the upper end of the ball of the thumb, just inside the inner border of the outer bone of the forearm, when the palm is forwards. It is felt with the tip of the middle finger, as it is theoretically possible to confuse one's own pulse if feeling with the thumb or index. The number of pulsations in a minute are counted and recorded.

Although the ancient Chinese are believed to have achieved great delicacy of diagnosis by taking the pulse, its use for our purpose will be confined to answering the two questions implied in the opening sentence above.

Should the second be in doubt, it must be decided whether the circumstances demand a search for the heartbeat at its site on the chest, just below the left breast. In most people it is easily felt with the flat of the hand.

Pus. The debris resulting from a battle between invading 'germs' and the body's defences. Usually creamy in colour and consistency, it is sometimes yellow or green; and may be blood-stained if bursting freshly from a boil or abscess, which is when it will most often be seen.

Pus should be allowed to discharge itself unless released by a doctor, and no attempt should be made to squeeze boils, etc, as this breaks the barrier which has been laid down between the diseased battle area and the surrounding tissues, and can result in widespread and serious infection.

Pus can spread infection. It should be gently removed on clean cotton wool which is then burnt, care being taken not to smear the pus on the skin.

Pyelitis (see *Kidney disease*).

Pyorrhoea. A chronic infection of the tooth sockets, leading to shrinking of the gums away from the teeth, infection of the underlying bone of the jaw, and eventual loosening of the teeth. Early recognition and treatment are important, and are matters for the dentist. (See *Gums*).

Quarantine. The length of time a patient suffering from, or who has been in contact with, infectious disease, should be kept away from others to whom he might spread it. The period and importance vary with the disease — eg, very important for whooping cough and young babies, and unimportant (by some opinion, inadvisable) for German measles and schoolgirls. Quarantine particulars are given for each disease mentioned herein.

Quinsy. Infection, usually one-sided, of the part of the throat surrounding the tonsil. It produces severe pain on swallowing and a characteristic throaty impediment of speech. The patient usually feels generally ill and should be seen by the doctor the same day, as early antibiotic treatment may be called for (**D**). Meanwhile, hot *isotonic saline* gargles every two hours, and *aspirin* or *paracetamol* tablets.

Rabies. A very dangerous disease transmitted by the bite of a dog or other mammal. The zone in which rabies is carried by foxes, squirrels, rats and bats is slowly spreading across Europe towards the Channel ports, and it will need only one mindlessly smuggled pet to bring it to the United Kingdom, which has been kept free for fifty years by the strict application of quarantine laws.

At present anyone bitten, scratched or licked by any animal outside Great Britain and Scandinavia, however mildly, should seek advice (**S**) or (**D**) as to whether a course of vaccination is necessary.

Rash. A temporary disturbance of the skin, usually involving 'spots' of varying size, shape, and distribution. A rash which disappears in a few hours is unlikely to be that of an infectious disease with the occasional exception of a mild attack of *German measles*.

Of the short duration rashes, *nettle rash* is the commonest, and is not infectious. Most rashes need medical diagnosis, and the question is whether to take the patient to the doctor's surgery or to ask the doctor to call, in case there may be infection. Clearly, if the patient is too ill to travel, there is no problem.

The following infectious diseases produce discoloration of the skin only, not lumps or blisters:

Scarlet fever. A very fine close rash, quickly spreading all over the body, which looks as if it had been dipped quickly in boiling water; the cheeks red, a white circle round the mouth. The patient is feverish and has often had a severe sore throat for one or two days. A milder form in which the patient is scarcely ill, is sometimes classed as a 'Toxic Rash'. In both cases (D or V).

Measles. Usually after four days or more of 'cold' symptoms and a remorseless dry cough, often with fever, a coarse blotchy rash appears behind the ears, and moves down the neck on to the body, darkening in hue, and the blotches occasionally running into each other. (V) unless condition of patient calls for an earlier visit.

German measles. The rash similar in form to that of measles but fainter, spreading in the same way; and little general illness. Although some of these find their way into doctors' waiting rooms by mistake, it is best to ask for a call (V), or telephone and describe the rash, before taking the patient to surgery.

The infectious disease with scattered small pink lumps, which blister in a day or two, is **chickenpox.** The rash of *shingles* carries the chickenpox infection; it is usually dealt with by surgery attendance unless for a particular reason. A rash which can mimic chickenpox is papular urticaria, with small raised red itching spots, usually in a scattered group on one or two sites on the body. Commonest in childhood, they are thought usually to be due to allergic reaction to animal fleas (cat, dog, or bird) or to outdoor insects such as grass mites. (V or S at doctor's direction.)

An irregular weepy rash on the face, often near the mouth and looking as if apricot jam had survived the last meal, is suspicious of *impetigo* (S).

Napkin rash (see under that heading). (See also *Eczema, Ringworm, Herpes.*)

Records, personal. Records should be kept for each member of the family, showing what *vaccinations* and immunizations they have had, with the dates; and the names and dates of any illnesses. These are often needed for applications for schools and employment, and when proposing for life assurance. A compact accessible home record, (see p. v) guards against the possibility of clerical breakdown, which has been known to occur, even in the best-run medical practices. See *Pregnancy* about recording menstrual dates.

Relaxation (see also *Pregnancy*). For our purpose, the practice of consciously relaxing tense muscles: **1** As a regular daily routine combined with a period of *contemplation*. **2** To prevent painful over-use of groups of muscles, particularly those concerned with the maintenance of posture.

1 There are many ways of doing it, and several good books dealing with the subject. Here is one idea. Calculate when in the day 10 to 20 minutes can most conveniently be spared, and fix on that time daily. Lie on your back on a firm mattress or several layers of blanket on a carpeted floor. A small pillow under the head, a folded bath towel as a pad in the hollow of the lower back. Allow the eyelids to close, as if by their own weight. The mind now undertakes a leisurely survey of the whole body, 'scanning' each part in turn, as a radar scans a landscape, and always returning to the head and neck as a starting and finishing point.

First, let the head sink into the pillow; feel the full weight of it being pulled downwards by gravity. Relax the muscles behind the neck — there is no question of *forcing* the head backwards, only *letting* it fall. Now turn attention to the arms, keeping the head still and relaxed. The upper arms rest on the mattress by the sides of the chest, the hands loosely flexed, palms downward, on the front of the thighs or lower abdomen. Attend first to the fingers, consciously loosening them, feel the weight of the palms and wrists collapsed against

THE SPINAL COLUMN

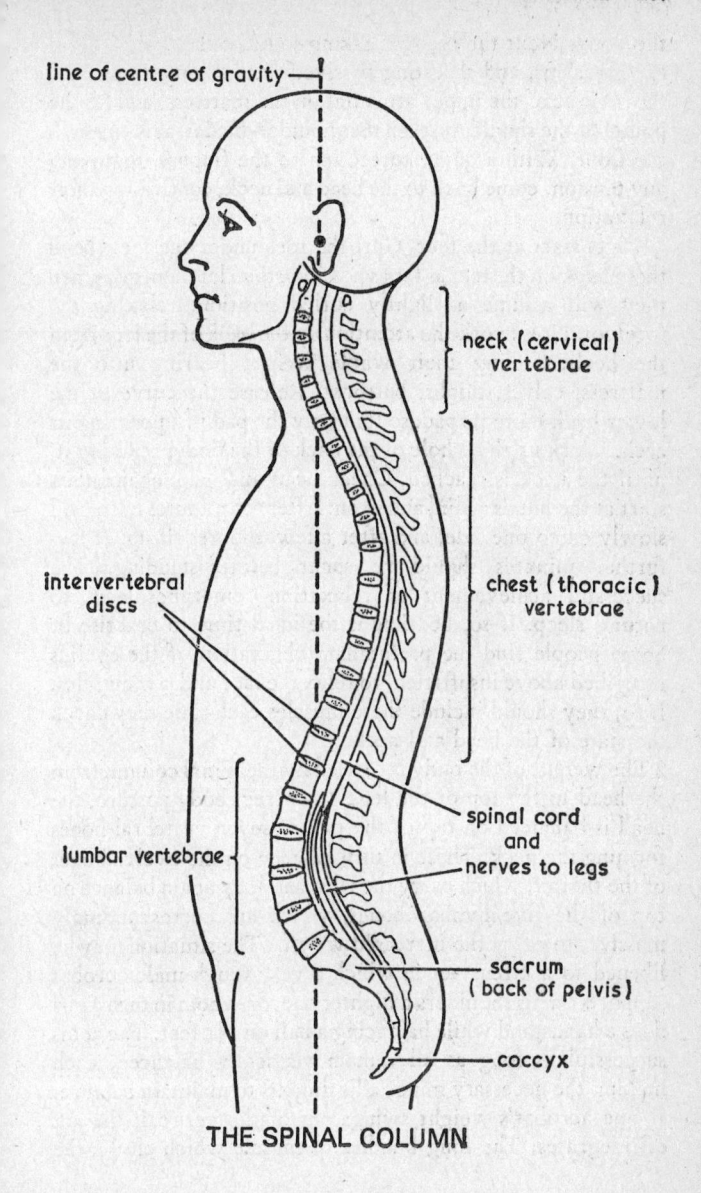

the body. Next the elbows, taking some of the weight from the forearms, and thrusting passively into the mattress. Feel the weight of the upper arms flat on the mattress, and let the points of the shoulders, then the shoulder-blades, sink towards the floor. With a quick correction to the fingers, removing any tension, come back to the head and neck, confirming their relaxation.

Next start at the feet. Curl the toes under the feet; bend them back on the feet as far as possible, then let them go, when they will assume a slightly curled position, relaxing the forefoot. Now work the attention up the back of the legs from the heels, feeling their whole weight bearing into the mattress; calves, thighs, buttocks. Release the curve of the lower back on to its pad, so that only the pad is supporting its arch. Work up the whole of the back of the body, relaxing it, until the neck is reached. Check head and neck again, then start at the hands again, and so on. After ten minutes or so, roll slowly on to one side, and after a few minutes sit up. A few further minutes should be spent before standing. The successful achievement of relaxation sometimes leads to natural sleep. If so, bedtime is the ideal time to practise it. Some people find the preliminary relaxation of the eyelids described above insufficient to relax the face and jaw muscles. If so, they should include these muscles each time they check the state of the head and neck.

2 The weight of the body is carried by the spinal column from the head to the top of the legs. In correct body posture, the head is balanced on top of the pile of seven vertebral bones forming the neck. These in turn balance on the twelve bones of the thorax, which carry the ribs, and they again balance on top of the five lumbar bones, which are correspondingly massive, to carry the increased weight. The situation may be likened to a circus act in which a very tough male acrobat supports on his shoulders a slighter one, on whom in turn a girl does a handstand while balancing a ball on her feet. The act is successful as long as all remain vertically balanced, each making the necessary minor adjustments to maintain balance. If one acrobat's weight swings out of the vertical, the act disintegrates. The long bundles of muscle which clothe the

spinal curves, front, back, and sides, are designed for short-term work. They give corrective tugs when the balance is threatened, or fix parts of the back firmly while strength is exerted by the limbs; but if, for instance, the head and neck are held persistently forward of the vertical position, in a 'peering' position, the muscles behind the neck are called on for continuous pulling to prevent the head falling forward. After a time they tire, release their load, and are made to contract again as the head tends to fall forwards. If continued, muscle fatigue results in loss of support for the joints of the neck bones, which then have to bear a load they were not designed for, and joint strain or deformity may eventually result. In the short-term, continuous stimulation of muscles already overtired leads to painful spasm in the muscles, most commonly experienced as headache — at the back when the neck muscles are affected, or in the temple if prolonged tension has fatigued the muscles which close the jaw. (See also *Motorist's leg*.)

The management of localized muscle tensions entails using the technique learned in general relaxation while other parts of the body remain active. Clearly no progress can be made with the spinal muscles until postural correction has relieved them of the need for continual contraction. The following simple routine will help. Stand with the back to a plain flat wall (no skirting board), the heels, buttocks, shoulders, and back of head touching the wall, knees straight. The lower back should be just sufficiently hollow to allow in the flat of the fingers. Attain your full height by reaching for the ceiling with the top of the head, not tilting it back. Spend about five minutes thus, *feeling* the head upwards as though it were a gas balloon, keeping the back of the head against the wall, and looking straight ahead as though into the eyes of someone your own height. Breathe in, swinging the upper ribs forward and upwards first, holding them up while the descending diaphragm relaxes the abdominal muscles. Breathe out by contracting the lower abdominal muscles first, squeezing the air out from below and relaxing the upper ribs last. It will often be found that these have been carried too low as part of a slumped posture and that when this is corrected, the upper ribs are held in a partly 'inflated' position. Now, spend a few minutes consciously relaxing the various muscles of the neck and shoulders, giving the feeling that the head is just balanced on top of the neck, ready to roll off in any direction. Last, take a few steps about the room keeping the posture as far as possible, always looking *out through the eyes*, and not peering *with the eyes*. Move the eyes to look downwards, don't move the head. After a few steps, return to the wall to check posture, then try again. Repeat the process two or three times a day. After a time it will be found that the correct posture of the head can be assumed at any time, and the muscles at the back and sides of the neck can then be allowed to relax, only giving an occasional pull to prevent the head rolling out of position. The benefit will be felt spreading to the shoulders, arms, and lower back.

Rheumatic Fever. One of the forms of acute rheumatism, rarer than it was twenty years ago. Children are most often affected. Typically, some ten to twenty days after a feverish sore throat which may have been recognized as *tonsillitis*, the patient becomes feverish and complains of joint or limb pains. The important thing is to recognize that the patient has slipped back after recovering from his first illness, and to keep him resting until the doctor can diagnose the cause (V). Have ready a *specimen of urine*, as the doctor may wish to exclude *kidney disease*, one form of which can also follow an infected throat at about the same interval.

If rheumatic fever is diagnosed, prolonged rest may be needed to avoid damage to the heart. After recovery, it is sometimes necessary to continue taking an antibiotic, to protect against further attacks. Sometimes rheumatic fever leaves the patient with a scarred heart valve, which may involve a reduction of activity. If so, the patient may be warned to avoid the extremes of physical exertion, and may also be warned always to inform dentist and doctor of his condition before teeth are extracted, so that antibiotic cover can be arranged.

A less severe form (sub-acute rheumatism) can continue for several months, giving rise to aching in the legs. Pains in the legs are sometimes called 'growing pains', a comfortable deception which should not be entertained; there are many causes of pains in the legs, but natural growth is not one of them, and the doctor should be consulted (**C**).

Rheumatic Fever, a handbook for Parents can be had free from the Arthritis and Rheumatism Council, through your doctor only. (Take him two stamped envelopes, a large one which should be addressed to yourself and a small one stamped only.) See *Arthritis* and also *St Vitus's Dance*.

Rheumatism. A wide term, indicating painful disability in the joints or the tissues associated with them. The joints themselves are covered under *Arthritis*. (See also *Spondylosis* and *Fibrositis*.)

Anyone handicapped by rheumatism (or other disability) should get in touch with the Social Services department of their local authority, to take advantage of the help available to disabled people. The Arthritis and Rheumatism Council publish *Your Home and Your Rheumatism*. This is available from the Council at 8–10 Charing Cross Road, London WC2H 0HN.

Acute rheumatism. A group of diseases affecting younger people. See *Rheumatic fever* and *St Vitus's Dance*.

Rhinitis (see under *Hay Fever*).

Ricked neck (see *Spondylosis*).

Rigor. An attack of shivering at the start of an acute illness, such as pneumonia. The patient feels cold and shivers uncontrollably, with teeth chattering. The *temperature* is usually about normal at the beginning (take in the armpit for five minutes), and rises during the attack. Wrap the patient in blankets until shivering ceases, after which only normal bedclothes coverage is needed. Give sips of warm drinks (tea, milk, soup, cocoa, etc) (**D**).

Rigor Mortis. The stiffening of the muscles of a corpse which starts within a few hours of death, first noticeable in the muscles controlling the jaw.

Ringworm and **Tinea.** An infection of the skin by a *fungus*. Scalp ringworm starts as a small red patch, slightly raised. The growing edge of fungus moves outwards, forming an irregular circle, raised at the edge (hence the name, but there is no worm). The hairs may be shed from inside the circle, where a bald patch with broken stumps of hair may be the first sign. It may be confused with *alopecia areata* and medical advice is needed, as also for the accurate diagnosis of patches on other parts of the skin (S).

Infection between the toes (*'athlete's foot'*) or in the groin ('dhobie itch') is common and can spread to toe and finger nails, and the nail folds (S). The infection can persist in shoes and games shorts, and can cause recurrences, so advice should be sought on disinfecting these.

Ringworm and Tinea can be started by sharing caps or other clothes that have been in contact with the affected skin. Domestic and farm animals are often infected, and attacks occur in farm workers by direct contact.

Rupture (hernia). The commonest form, inguinal hernia, is a smooth swelling in the groin extending towards the genital area, and sometimes in the male reaching the *scrotum*. It needs either surgical repair or the constant wearing of a truss or belt, to keep the swelling from protruding. The appliance is put on before getting out of bed, and taken off on lying down at night. A rupture which escapes from the control of the truss is in danger of strangulation. That is, it becomes fixed in the groin or scrotum and cannot be returned to the abdomen by *gentle* pressure when the patient lies down with his head relaxed on a pillow. A patient who knows he has a rupture will usually know how to ease it back by gently manipulating with the fingers. No attempt at pushing it back should be made, and no one other than the patient should try to return it. If there is any reason to suspect strangulation (the patient often vomits copiously), or if there is pain after replacement, or the patient's condition deteriorates, the doctor must be sent for (U). The doctor should be consulted (S) when a rupture is first discovered or suspected.

St Vitus's Dance (Chorea). One of the forms of acute rheumatism, characterized by spasmodic movements of the face, hands and arms; sometimes of the whole body. They differ from a 'tic' in being random, whereas the movements of a tic repeat themselves. The severity of the movements and the degree of nervous disturbance accompanying them varies. Early diagnosis and treatment (which may involve several weeks' rest) are important in minimizing the occurrence of heart trouble, which can complicate this, as other types of acute rheumatism (S or V according to severity). (See *Rheumatic fever.*)

Scabies. An infectious skin disease, usually spread by close contact, and giving rise to intense itching. The hands and fingers are usually involved first, and very small blisters together with short 'runs' like pin scratches, may be seen. It is caused by a mite too small to be seen by the naked eye. Once diagnosed, it can be successfully treated, provided the instructions given are carried out completely, but diagnosis is not always easy, and confusion with certain allergic disorders is possible (C).

Scalds (see *Burns*).

Scarlet Fever. A form of acute *tonsillitis* in which poisons released by the infecting streptococcus (see *Germs*) cause a finely stippled red rash on trunk and limbs, usually on the second day of the illness. The *temperature* is high, 38.5 to 40°C (101 to 104°F), the throat sore, and the glands behind the angle of the jaw tender and swollen. It is a notifiable infectious disease, and the doctor should be asked to call (D or V).

In the weeks after the illness, the skin of the palms and the soles often flakes off. It used to be thought that the flakes could carry the disease, but this is not so.

A similar illness of mild form is sometimes known as 'toxic rash'. An occasional complication, as of other forms of tonsillitis, is acute *nephritis*, and anyone who develops puffy eyes or ankles ten days or so after an attack, or whose urinary output drops significantly, should have medical attention (V). Another rare complication is *rheumatic fever.*

Quarantine for the patient is three weeks, or longer if there are complications. Adult contacts engaged in preparing or serving food should not work until cleared by the Community Physician. Child contacts are not usually excluded from school. Incubation period 2 to 5 days.

Schizophrenia. A group of mental disorders with widely differing symptoms, and of serious national and personal importance. Nationally, 1 per cent of the population suffers at some time from some form of schizophrenia, a fact which would be more obvious had not so many patients become permanent residents in mental hospitals before the recent advances in treatment.

The popular phrase 'split mind' does not give a good idea of the disease. 'Disintegrated mind' would be nearer the truth, for patients may show defects in any or all aspects of mental activity. Early signs are failure of concentration, which the patient may notice and complain of, vagueness and inability to develop an argument or explanation, loss of normal emotional relationship with those close to him, increasing apathy, self-neglect, and ill-temper. To some extent, these defects are to be found at times in normally developing adolescents, and as three quarters of all cases of schizophrenia start between the ages of 15 and 25, it can be difficult to know where adolescent difficulty ends and mental illness begins. A *sudden* increase in vagueness and apathy should alert those about the patient, and suggest a medical opinion. If possible, the doctor should be given a compact account of the situation before he sees the patient.

Cases starting in the late twenties are more likely to be physically violent, and may become dangerous if delusions and hallucinations set them against others. If violence threatens, retreat in good time and call help from neighbours, police, doctor, or ambulance department. Compulsory admission to hospital may be necessary, and the appropriate Social Worker will then be called by police or doctor (see *Insanity*).

Delusions and hallucinations are prominent if the disease starts in the thirties or later, and these sometimes bring the patient into conflict with authority.

Schizophrenia remains a very serious mental illness in spite of the recent improvements in treatment, and by no means all patients can be expected to recover completely. When improvement follows the use of drugs, these often need to be continued for many years, and members of the patient's family can help him by encouraging him in this, as the tendency to omit or reduce doses is very common.

Sciatica. Pain felt in the buttock, back of thigh, calf and/or ankle, made worse on flexing the thigh with the knee straight (gently!). It is not a disease, but the name of a pain which has many causes. The commonest is pressure on the sciatic nerve by a prolapsed lumbar disc (see *Lumbago*), but all cases of sciatica need medical help (**S** or **V**).

Screening Tests. Tests applied to a group or a whole population in the hope of detecting early certain diseases of which the victims are unaware. An example of a test available to the whole population is the mass X-ray for detection of diseases of the chest. Others are:

1 The Mantoux test for *tuberculosis*, offered to all children in local authority secondary schools (and in private schools by arrangement with the Community Physician).
2 Phenylketonuria test carried out on newborn babies to pick out the rare cases of a disorder of body chemistry needing a special diet throughout childhood.

Not yet organized on a large scale is a urine test for unsuspected *diabetes*. It is a simple one, and could be carried out by family doctors and health visitors, but they would be swamped, unless it could be properly organized. Time could be found in most practices to check a *specimen of urine* passed two or three hours after a starchy meal (bread, potatoes, cereal), from people at greater than average risk, that is, close relatives of diabetics, and people who are overweight.

Spina bifida. By the time this is printed, there should be firm information about the feasibility of the test, performed in pregnancy, for the recognition of spinal deformity.

The Cervical Smear test, for early detection of the threat of cancer of the neck of the womb, is now widely available. One should be clear that this tests only the *neck* (cervix) (see p.162 for illustration), and not be misled into neglecting signs from the body of the womb, particularly irregular bleeding (see *Menstruation* and *Menopause*).

The scarcity of skilled workers restricts screening for *glaucoma* to the eye departments of some larger hospitals. Some ophthalmic specialists advise that this test should eventually form part of the routine examination of the eyes for everyone over 40, with priority to those who have a family history of glaucoma.

One of the simplest screening tests of all is carried out by the patient at regular intervals of one to three months, soon after the menstrual 'period'. This is the search of the female breasts for *lumps*. The breasts should be thoroughly felt over at bath time, the search extending up to the armpits, and should be viewed face-on in a mirror with the arms raised above the head — a position which may bring to light any lack of symmetry caused by deep inflammation. Any discovery is reported to the doctor (S). Of course, these examinations should continue after the menopause. An instruction leaflet is often obtainable from one's local clinic or health centre.

Scrotum. The scrotum is the bag or purse containing the male genital organs (testicles). The commonest cause of painful swelling is inflammation of a testicle (orchitis), which occurs most frequently in *mumps*, but can follow inflammation or operation on the bladder and *prostate* gland. It usually produces fever and general illness, confining the patient to bed (D).

Pain and tenderness starting suddenly in a testicle, often after a twist or blow, or on sitting down awkwardly, may be due to the organ becoming twisted, interfering with its blood supply, and needs medical aid the same day (D or S).

A painless swelling feeling like a small bag of worms in one side of the scrotum is a varicocele (group of enlarged veins) and is not usually of any importance, though the doctor should be consulted when it is first noticed (C).

A smooth swelling, usually painless, extending from the

groin downwards towards the testicle is a *rupture* (hernia). A similar smooth soft swelling confined to the scrotum and not connected with the groin is usually due to a collection of fluid called a hydrocele. It is more often seen in older men, is not serious, and can be treated satisfactorily by the doctor or surgeon (C). Any swelling found in the scrotum should be seen by the doctor for accurate diagnosis (C). (See also *Testicle*).

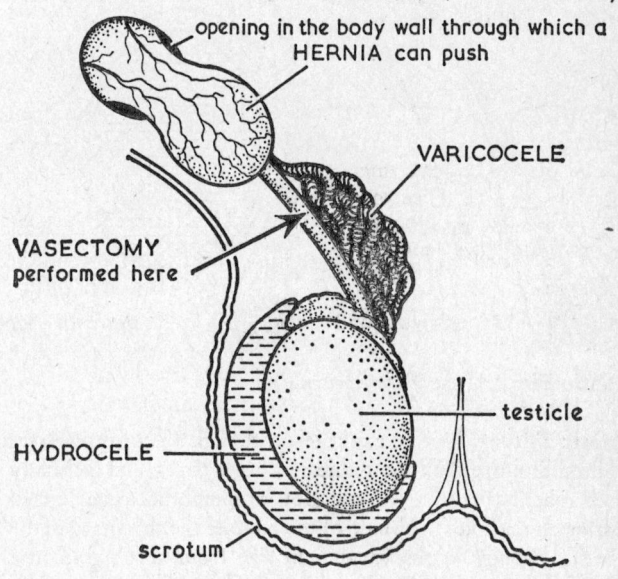

Sea Sickness (see *Travel Sickness*).

Sebaceous Cyst. Results from a blockage of one of the tiny sebaceous glands of the skin, which make and secrete protective grease on to the hair, as it grows out of the skin. The continuing production of grease causes the blocked gland to swell into a cyst, which bulges above the surface of the skin. The size of a pea when first noticed, it can grow to that of a golf ball, though if it is on the scalp (a common site) the patient will usually demand its removal before that. Removal is by a minor operation. (See illustration, p. 218.)

A sebaceous cyst which becomes painful, hot, red, and tender to touch, is infected, and should be seen by the doctor (**S**). Meanwhile, the pain will be relieved by *hot packs*. (See also *Lump, Cyst*.)

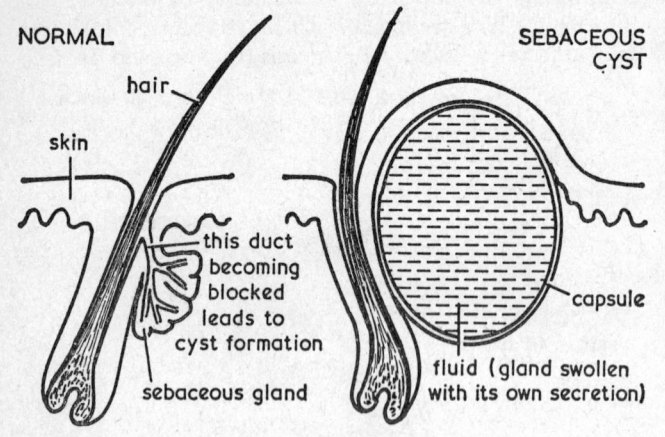

NORMAL — hair, skin, this duct becoming blocked leads to cyst formation, sebaceous gland

SEBACEOUS CYST — capsule, fluid (gland swollen with its own secretion)

Septic Finger (see *Finger, poisoned*).

Septic Throat. Not an exact term, though a descriptive one. It implies more than the redness of a *sore throat*, and is usually used when creamy or yellow spots or membranes can be seen either on the folds each side of the back of the throat, or in the tonsils; spongy knobs varying in size from an almond to a walnut, lying within those folds. Commonly caused by *tonsillitis*, Vincent's infection (see *Gums*), and in times past, diphtheria. Should diphtheria become active again, the old precaution of keeping a patient who shows 'membrane' in the throat resting completely until seen by a doctor should be observed (**D**). Other cases should be treated on their merits — if patient is ill and feverish (**D** or **V**, if not **S**). Meanwhile, keep his crockery and cutlery separate.

Shingles (see *Herpes zoster*).

Shock. A person 'suffering from shock' after an accident is usually suffering from being shaken and frightened. In the absence of injury, a cup of tea and a rest in a warm room is usually all that he needs. True shock is a more serious business, and is caused by severe burns or loss of blood, either externally, or internally by bleeding into damaged tissues. It is made worse by rough handling, exposure to cold, and delay in reaching a casualty department equipped for blood transfusion. Avoidance consists in:

1. Stopping *bleeding*,
2. Immediate summoning of ambulance or qualified first aid, meanwhile
3. Minimum movements needed to place patient out of danger.
4. Maintenance of body heat by blankets etc, but no artificial heating.
5. Comfort and reassurance.
   Giving anything by mouth is best avoided if there is any possibility of an anaesthetic being needed in the course of the next 4 hours. (But see under *Burns* for fluid requirements during transport to hospital.)

See also *Injuries, Bleeding, Burns,* and *Scalds*.

Shoplifting. Some cases constitute serious social accidents, for which no ordinary reason can be found. More women than men are involved, probably because more women than men shop, and men carry no handbags — virtue doesn't enter into it. Unexplained shoplifting is a particular risk at the time of the menopause, and when younger women are overstressed with the care of young children, insufficient time, and marital or financial worry. Most of it happens in self-service stores, and some precautions should be observed.

1. Make a shopping list before starting out.
2. Do self-service shopping first in the day, when shopping bags or baskets are empty. If at all possible, leave these at the store entrance and put all purchases in the store's container.
3. Do not open your bag or purse until you reach the pay desk.

4 Do not shop self-service when you are pressed for time, are likely to be distracted by children, or have something weighing on your mind.

Sight. Anyone who notices any alteration in their sight, by day or night, should see a doctor or optician as soon as possible. Irrevocable harm can occur while one delays in the belief that one's 'glasses need changing'. They probably do, but meanwhile an unsuspected *glaucoma* could damage the sight permanently. (See *Screening tests, Glaucoma*.) Sudden loss or alteration of sight needs help urgently. If a doctor cannot see it at once, get yourself to the nearest Accident and Emergency Department of a hospital at all speed; in some conditions, every half-hour counts.

Sinus and **Sinusitis.** A number of caves open out of the inside of the nose, and though strictly these are all called sinuses, the word 'sinus' usually means the frontal sinus, which lies in the bone of the forehead between, and above, the eyes. It communicates with the topmost part of the nose by a narrow passage. Below each eye, the hollow cheekbone on each side contains the antrum (plural 'antra') and these also communicate with the nose. The lining membrane of the nose and breathing tubes, with its protecting coat of sticky mucus, continues into these caves, the mucus formed in them draining back into the nose and washing out any germs which may have penetrated. An attack of sinusitis or antritis occurs if the lining membrane of the nose becomes so swollen, by common cold or hay fever for instance, that the passage to the sinus is blocked. Mucus accumulates and becomes infected, causing pain which can be severe.

Many mild cases respond to *steam inhalations* repeated two hourly, followed by the use of ephedrine nasal drops, if they are available. (For method see *Pain in Head*.) If pain is severe or increasing, or if the temperature is rising, the doctor is needed (**S** or **D**). Meanwhile, *aspirin* or *paracetamol* tablets will help a little. Sleeping with the head of the bed tilted up about 6 inches will reduce the pain often felt on waking.

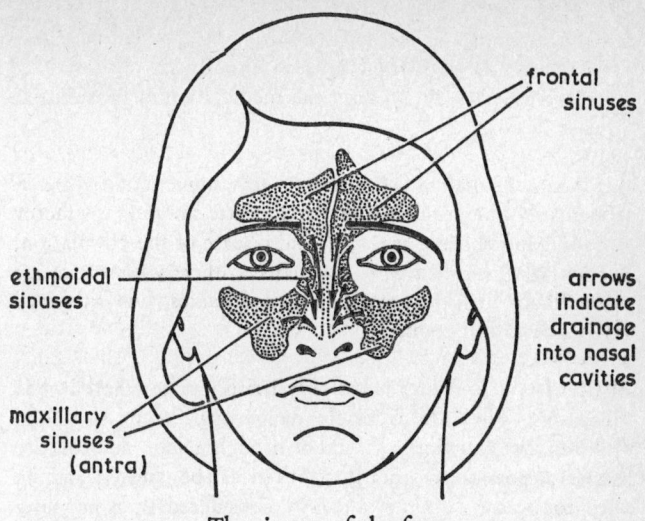

The sinuses of the face — frontal sinuses; ethmoidal sinuses; maxillary sinuses (antra); arrows indicate drainage into nasal cavities

Sleeplessness (see *Insomnia*).

Sling (see illustration on p. 151).

Smallpox. A serious illness caused by a virus, not normally present in this country. Outbreaks can occur rapidly if introduced from abroad by travellers; particularly air travellers, who may complete their journey between exposure to infection abroad and developing the disease themselves. Protection is by vaccination, producing an attack of cowpox, a much milder related disease, introduced through a scratch on the skin. If this produces a cowpox sore, the body organizes protection which covers the related disease of smallpox. Vaccination, which is no longer compulsory in this country, is done by the patient's general practitioner, who should be given three or four days' notice to allow him to obtain the necessary material. *Anyone with eczema should not be vaccinated* unless for special reasons, and the doctor should always be told beforehand if there is a history of *eczema, dermatitis, nettle rash* or urticaria in the patient or any of his near relatives.

See also under *Vaccination*.
Incubation Period: 10 to 17 days, usually 12.
Quarantine: as directed by the medical authorities, but at least 17 days.

Smoking. As well as favouring the development of *lung cancer*, it seems that moderate or heavy cigarette smoking is a factor in producing chronic *bronchitis*, and disease of the circulation, particularly *coronary disease*. Pregnant mothers who smoke are more likely to have growth-retarded babies, with lowered resistance to infection.

Snakebite. The Adder is the only British snake whose bite is poisonous. The bite is rarely dangerous except to young children, but any victim should be brought under medical care as soon as possible in order that the risk can be assessed, and the need for serum administration be considered. It is not now considered necessary to apply a tourniquet, nor to cut or suck the wound.

Often mistaken for an Adder is the Smooth Snake, a harmless inhabitant of southern England, and since 1975 protected by Act of Parliament. It is not therefore practicable to kill an offending snake for identification, and one must rely on a knowledge of differences in appearance.

Adders average 20 in. in length and live in or near woodland. Older females may be up to 30 in. long. The colour varies, but they all have a *continuous* dark zigzag line down their backs. The Smooth Snake favours dry country, is up to 20 in. long, and has *separate* dark spots down its back. The harmless Grass Snake lives in damp areas, is up to 3 ft long, has a yellow mark either side of its head, and a much less obvious pattern on its back.

Should anyone be close enough, an inspection of the eyes is infallible. The Adder has a vertical slit pupil, the Smooth Snake's is round.

Snoring. A lot of people snore when they sleep on their backs. They sometimes do this because they have backache, and it is worth trying two *aspirin* or *paracetamol* tablets at night, combined with a cord tied round the waist with a cotton reel at the back. Tilting the head end of the bed four to seven inches may help. Of course, there are many other causes, and one should not be too fatalistic — an ear, nose and throat specialist may be able to help, and some family doctors have a special interest in the subject (C).

Sore Throat. The ordinary sore throat often associated with the start of a cold is pharyngitis, or faucitis. On looking at the back of the mouth in a mirror, the sides, wall, and roof of the throat are engorged, showing dark red. The uvula — little finger of flesh hanging from the top of the arch — may be swollen and give rise to irritation when it interferes with swallowing. Best treated with *aspirin* or *paracetamol* tablets, 2 every 4 or 5 hours for adults — children's doses under *Aspirin* and *Paracetamol* — and plentiful drinks of all kinds. (See also *Quinsy, Septic throat, Tonsillitis.*)

Spastic. Originally, an ajective used to describe a condition of continual spasm in a muscle, due to faulty messages reaching it from injured brain cells. It is now applied to victims of brain damage — usually caused at birth — resulting in one or more limbs being crippled by spastic muscles, and is loosely used of sufferers from other types of brain injury.

Parents suffering the shock of discovering that they have a 'spastic' baby, should get in touch with the nearest branch of the Spastics Society (Telephone Directory, or through the London Headquarters, 12 Park Crescent, London W1N 4EQ) for help of every kind. Send a stamped addressed envelope.

Specimen of Urine. Your doctor may wish to examine the urine, and will then ask you to bring a 'specimen' of it. If possible, let this be the first urine passed in the day; about two ounces in a clean bottle with your name on the label. If you are complaining of pain on passing water, excessive thirst, swelling of the feet or ankles, or if the urine passed seems to contain blood or looks unusual, take a specimen of it with you, without waiting to be asked (S). Sometimes, a special collection technique is used — the doctor or his nurse will advise if this is needed.

Splinter, removal of. If there is enough of a splinter sticking out of the skin, removal is simple. Sterilize a pair of eyebrow tweezers, or similar tool, by boiling it for five or ten minutes. Grasp the end of the splinter and pull it out. A splinter below the skin's surface should not be interfered with, unless it can be removed by an old countryman's trick described in the *British Medical Journal* by Dr David Langley. A narrow-necked bottle is filled with hot water and emptied when the glass is as hot as possible. The neck of the bottle is then placed over the splinter and, as the bottle cools, suction is exerted on it. The bottle may need to be heated and reapplied several times before the splinter is drawn out.

If neither of these methods serves, it is best to see the doctor during the first 24 hours (S). Once a splinter has been extracted *hot bathing* should be continued every 4 hours for 48 hours. If the splinter wound becomes painful, throbbing, red, or swollen, or if the splinter may have been contaminated with road dirt, manure, or soil, (S) in order that antibiotic or antitetanus treatment may be considered.

Spondylosis. The name at present used for a common and variable disorder of the joints of the spine, responsible for some cases of stiff neck ('fibrositis'), *neuralgia* in the chest, *lumbago*, and *sciatica*; also occasionally *vertigo* or *fainting*. Speaking broadly, the spine consists of 24 'vertebrae', each consisting of a body like a cotton reel, to the back of which a bony arch is attached. Strung together, the arches form a long bony tube through which passes the spinal cord, carrying the nerve 'cables' from the brain, and some of the main arteries supplying blood to the brain. The vertebrae are hooked on to each other by two small joints at each end, so that the whole spine is flexible, and between each vertebral body is a hydraulic shock-absorbing disc, consisting of a jelly centre contained in a tough capsule.

It seems that in early adult life some of these discs can lose their elasticity, and a sudden strain or prolonged pressure, as by sleeping with the neck crooked, can squeeze them out of shape, so that the movement of the spine is locked and nerves or blood vessels may be pressed on. The commonest result is a stiff neck, with movement restricted on turning or bending the head to one or other side. It is sometimes complicated by *vertigo* or double vision, and these conditions will need a doctor's help (**S** or **D**). An uncomplicated stiff neck can result from a locked joint, and will often clear on its own in a few days, using *aspirin*, *paracetamol*, a guarded *hot water bottle* for ten minutes every few hours, and a *butterfly pillow* at night. If it does not, or if the condition is severe, consult the doctor (**S**). The term 'spondylosis' can more accurately be applied when a number of discs have shrunk or altered shape, allowing the vertebrae which they had held separate to come closer together, so that their joints over-engage. This reduces the apertures through which nerves and arteries pass, and also gives rise to diffuse painful stiffness, to which the general terms fibrositis or muscular rheumatism have been applied. Pain may extend to the shoulders and arms, if the neck bones are affected. The treatment is long-term, and may involve postural re-education, physiotherapy, and exercises (**C**). (See also *Disc, Slipped; Lumbago* and *Posture*.)

Sprain. Occurs when a joint is accidentally forced beyond its normal range of movement, so that one or more of the ligaments (fibrous cords anchoring the bones to each other across the joint) are weakened, torn, or pulled out of their attachment to the bone. The ligaments are not suited to taking sudden strains, a job usually done by the muscles controlling the joint, and a sprain results when the muscles have been 'taken off guard' by the rapidity of the movement. Thus, when climbing stairs, the muscles holding the foot straight on the ankle will relax when the foot feels the step, ready for another group to take over and raise the body weight on to the toes. Should it prove that the foot has not a good hold on the step, or should the carpet slip, the foot will slip back to the previous step, and if the climb has been made sideways-on, the outside of the slipped foot will double under, lacking muscular control. The whole body weight will contribute to this movement and the ankle joint will roll outwards over the outer edge of the foot, tearing the corresponding ligament or even cracking the end of the fibula bone which forms the outside of the ankle hinge. The first stage constitutes a sprained ankle, the commonest sprain encountered. At the time it happens, or shortly afterwards, it is acutely painful and the patient may feel sick or even faint. In the latter event he should be laid down, as shown on p. 247, when colour and consciousness will soon return. Advantage can be taken of the short period of unconsciousness by anyone sufficiently resolute to remove the footwear before the ankle swells, as it

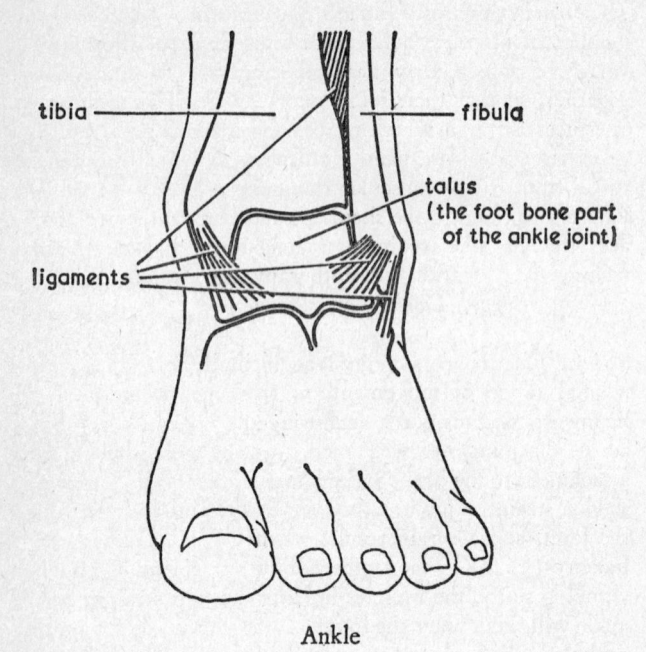

Ankle

(labels: tibia, fibula, talus (the foot bone part of the ankle joint), ligaments)

soon will. Pain will be lessened if the foot is propped up — support the whole leg from heel to thigh; do not let the knee bridge the gap between a stool and a chair. The patient can be given a warm drink and two or three *aspirin* or *paracetamol*

- If a patient is not within the scope of home care, or worsens in spite of it, or if there is any uncertainty, a doctor should be consulted.

tablets while a trained first aid worker is sought, or arrangements made to transport him to doctor or Casualty Department. This is advisable in all but the mildest sprains, as an X-ray may be needed to exclude broken bones. In the first few hours, a *cold pack* relieves pain. There is a tendency for an ankle which has once been sprained to repeat the process more easily on subsequent twists — or perhaps it was more 'sprainable' from the beginning. Anyway, it is wise to protect the ankle when playing, climbing, etc, by wearing a crepe bandage applied as a figure-of-eight round ankle and foot, and to wear walking or games boots where possible. Fatigue of muscles in the course of a long walk may allow a stumble to be converted into a sprain, and a boot allows just sufficient delay for the muscles to catch up on the situation.

Sputum (see *Phlegm*).

Squint. Lack of balance in the muscles which move the eyes, so that only one eye looks at an object, the other appearing to look elsewhere. It is important that treatment should start as early in life as possible, and the doctor should be consulted if a squint is suspected, even during the first year of life (C). If not treated, the patient will use only one eye, ignoring the vision of the squinting eye, which eventually becomes useless, so that the squinter is for practical purposes one-eyed, with poor judgement of distance, among other handicaps.

Stammer. Symptom of an emotional or nervous disturbance. It calls for expert assessment and treatment (C), and for an atmosphere of calm, sympathetic understanding from those around. It cannot be scolded, scorned, or punished away, and those in charge of other children should exert themselves to ensure that the victim is not teased about it.

Steam Inhalation. Used in the treatment of *common cold*, *sinusitis*, and laryngitis (*loss of voice*). The best known is Friars' Balsam, or Benzoin Inhalation BPC, but the inhalation of menthol and eucalyptus of the British National Formulary is sometimes more acceptable. A 5 ml spoonful of either is put in a jar and a pint of water just below boiling point is added. The stream is breathed in and out for five to ten minutes, the head and jar being enclosed in a 'tent' of bathtowel. Obviously, for a cold and sinusitis, the steam is taken in through the nose, for laryngitis through the mouth. The treatment is repeated every two to four hours. Keep the jar on a tray, in case of a spill.

Sterility. Failure to produce offspring although intercourse is normal. The cause may lie in either partner; the male may not be producing sperm, or producing them in insufficient numbers; or the sperm may not be able to reach the egg in the female, owing to obstruction of part of her genital pathway. Sometimes the female may not be producing eggs at all. In partners of average age, it is usual to allow two years of intercourse before investigating possible sterility, as many marriages will be fruitful during the second year. If partners are older at marriage, advice should be sought earlier in the hope of achieving pregnancies before increasing age makes child bearing and rearing more difficult. All cases require expert investigation, and the approach in the first instance should be to the family doctor (C). It often happens that no cause can be found, and the easing of tension produced by the knowledge that neither partner is sterile may then allow conception to take place. A similar happy consequence sometimes follows the decision to adopt a baby; it is not uncommon for the first pregnancy to start while overtures are being made to adoption societies. See also *Testicles*.

Steroids. Potent chemicals used in the treatment of serious diseases, often for months or years on end. Patients should carry a Steroid Card, with particulars of dosage, which they should always show to any doctor they see. Steroid treatment should never be stopped except on medical advice.

Stiff Neck (see *Spondylosis*).

Stings, 1 Insect. Chiefly from bees and wasps. They do not often become infected, and the pain and irritation settle in the course of a few hours. If the bee has left its sting in the skin, it should be gently removed with the edge of a knife, without squeezing it. *Cold compresses*, spirit or Eau de Cologne, can be applied to the skin, and *aspirin* or *paracetamol* tablets used to relieve the pain. A sting inside the mouth may lead to swelling of the throat or tongue. Sucking ice, and a *cold compress* round the throat will help while the patient is being taken to hospital. This should be done with all speed, in case breathing becomes obstructed.

A few people are allergic to bee or wasp stings, and if by chance the sting penetrates a small vein, the poison quickly sets up a severe reaction, with widespread *nettle rash*, difficult breathing, and swelling of lips, mouth, and throat. This is an emergency, and the patient should be brought under medical care in as few minutes as possible. When first stung, he should be asked if he carries any antidote, and if so, this should be given him. If he does not, inquire among the bystanders for any asthmatic or hay-fever subject, who may have adrenaline injections, an adrenaline or similar inhaler, or antihistamine tablets. If so, they should be given to the patient in the dose which their owner normally uses, but halved or quartered as necessary for children.

A patient who finds that he is allergic to stings — a patch of nettle rash round a sting may show that sensitivity is developing, or it may produce symptoms of *asthma* or *hay fever* — should consult his doctor for provision of a suitable antidote, which should then always be carried, and which should have clear instructions for use on the outside of the packet. The doctor will advise on the suitability of immunizing injections, which have recently been developed. *Anybody stung whose mouth or tongue becomes swollen should be brought under medical care forthwith.* Time spent waiting to see if it gets worse may be the only time available for safe transport. If hospital and doctor are within the same range of availability, choose the hospital, as facilities for inserting a breathing tube will be available, should it be needed.

A sting becoming increasingly red and tender some twelve hours or more after infliction, is probably infected and needs medical care (**S**). Meanwhile apply *hot packs*.

2 Stings while bathing.

(a) Jelly fish. The ordinary jelly fish encountered in European

waters cause burning pain and weals at the point of contact; and in the course of the next hour or so general symptoms of tightness in the chest and difficulty in breathing, with faintness and occasionally collapse may occur. For that reason it is wise to bring a patient who has been stung under medical supervision as soon as possible, so that any developments can be dealt with. The stung part should be gently wiped with water and sand as soon as possible, to remove any parts of the jelly fish still adhering, and if any antihistamine or hydrocortisone cream or lotion is available, it should be applied. Similarly, it sometimes happens that a bystander has antihistamine tablets to take for hay fever. These should be given in the dose directed on the package, halved or quartered if necessary for an older or young child. Lacking any of these, calamine lotion is often available and should be applied every quarter of an hour to the stung part. These measures are much more important if the sting is from a *Portuguese Man-of-War*. These occasionally reach western and southern waters of the United Kingdom in warm summers. They consist of inflated bladders which float on the surface trailing poisonous tentacles, which may be feet long in large speciments. On contact, the tentacle threads immediately sink into the skin and can't be brushed off, but the minute capsule of poison remain on the surface and should be washed off with wet sand and water at once. The general effects can be severe, and as they may start within ten minutes of the sting, every effort should be made to get the patient to hospital or doctor at once. In bad cases, the full resources of a hospital may be needed. Further to the measures described under jelly fish stings, any available antihistamine should be given in the dose written on the package (halved or quartered for children, as above) and any available asthmatic patient who has adrenaline injections, tablets for putting under his tongue, or an inhaler, should be asked to accompany the patient to hospital and to give him whichever of these treatments he has available (in the above order of preference) should he develop signs of difficulty in breathing.

(b) *Weever fish,* also called Bishop fish, usually lie in the sand near or below the low water mark, with only the dorsal fin exposed. If trodden on, its poisonous spines produce very painful stings, sometimes collapse and *shock*. As the venom is destroyed by heat, the treatment is to immerse the stung part in water as hot as can be tolerated without scalding. This is continued for from 30 to 90 minutes. Afterwards a clean dressing is applied, and if the injury is on the foot, the leg is kept up for 2 or 3 days. To be effective, the hot water treatment must start within 30 minutes. In some South West English resorts, the local doctors see numbers of these strings, and have evolved a treatment by injection which rapidly relieves the effects, if done within a short time of the sting. Cases of collapse or shock will in any case need doctor's help as soon as possible (UU).

3 Nettles. The stings last for a few hours only, and are relieved by *cold compresses*, calamine lotion, or spirit lotions. Nettle stings have nothing to do with *nettle rash*.

Stroke. The result of a 'cerebrovascular accident' in which interference with its circulation renders part of the brain temporarily or permanently inactive. Usually of sudden onset, it is more frequent after middle-age than before. Typically, the patient becomes unconscious, with face congested, one or more limbs may shake convulsively, and the bladder or bowel may empty. Breathing is deep and stertorous and one side of the mouth may be seen to be flabby. Saliva may dribble from the mouth, sometimes blood also if the tongue or lip has been injured in falling, or bitten; and the first task is to turn the head so that these fluids run out of the mouth and are not drawn into the lungs. At the same time, test the fit of the dentures, and if they are loose, remove them, though the patient may breathe more easily if well-fitting dentures are left in position. If the doctor is expected in the course of an hour or two, the patient may be made comfortable where he has fallen, with blankets and a thin pillow. If the site is not suited for this, movement may be undertaken to a mattress placed nearby, after making sure that there are no obvious broken bones, as might be shown by limbs or spine lying at an unnatural angle (see *Injuries*). If three lifters can be procured, the head, body, and legs can be moved in one piece. Look out for a trailing flaccid arm which may become caught in a doorway. The period of unconsciousness varies from a few seconds to a permanency, but many cases recover in the course of minutes rather than hours. If possible, they should be watched until consciousness returns, and preferably by someone they know. The watcher should try to imagine himself in the victim's place. He will wake knowing nothing of his attack, to find himself unable to move one side of his body, perhaps unable to speak, perhaps having fouled himself and almost certainly frightened. HE WILL NOT BE DEAF. In a quiet voice he should be told that he has had some sort of a fainting attack, that the doctor has been sent for, and that he should rest until he comes. If it has become apparent that the clothes are fouled, it should be intimated tactfully that one is aware of this, and a start may be made on removing clothes and cleansing, unless it is evident that the movements cause pain. If the patient obviously cannot speak, establish communication by asking him to wink once for yes, twice for no, or if he has good movement of a hand, to nod or shake the hand as it lies on the covers. Then ask has he any pain. If yes, go through the parts of the body, asking yes or no. If it is possible to examine the site complained of, do so — he may be lying on his pipe or a bunch of keys. If he is a stranger, ask if there is anyone you can get in touch with. If yes, ask in turn: Mr?, Mrs?, Miss? Then ask him to spell the surname, etc. One can go through the alphabet asking him to signal the right letter when you say it, but it is quicker to write an alphabet as a square with five letters on each side, A B C D E along the top, and A F K P U down the lefthand side. Ask him to wink or tap the number of the line, and then the number of the letter in it; or point to each line and column in turn. Make sure he has his spectacles if he needs them.

Next ask if he needs to pass water. If yes, a man can usually be arranged suitable with a jam jar or wide-mouthed bottle. A woman, lacking a bedpan, should be packed with three or four sanitary towels or wadding, the bed being protected with polythene or rubber sheet: but see *Injuries, Pelvis*.

The stroke may have made swallowing difficult. If the patient is thirsty, the corner of a clean cloth should be soaked in water and put in the mouth so that a few drops at a time can be sucked out of it. If that is successful, a feeding cup or teaspoon may be used, but very cautiously at first, to avoid risk of choking.

The severity of a stroke, degree of recovery, and the time it takes, vary greatly. A lot depends on morale and previous physical condition, but it is reasonable to assure a previously healthy patient that he can expect considerable recovery of activity. The doctor will decide whether the patient needs early hospital care or would be better under home conditions at first. Depending on what is available locally, he will advise about specialist rehabilitation.

Styes. Specialized boils affecting the sockets from which eyelashes grow. They may come in crops and are usually caused by *germs* carried by the finger, and rubbed into the edges of the lids. The two commonest reservoirs for germs are the nostrils and the fold between the buttocks. The belief that the victim of styes may need glasses arises from the fact that eyes are more likely to be rubbed if the sight is not correct. Individual styes are treated with packs wrung out of hot *isotonic saline* applied to the closed eyelids for ten minutes every four hours. If a bead of *pus* forms at the edge of the lid, surrounding an eyelash, the lash can be plucked with tweezers, allowing the pus to escape. The doctor should be consulted (**C**) about recurring styes so that any reservoir of infection can be treated.

Sunburn. The result of over-exposure of the skin to sunlight — either direct sunshine or reflected from water or low cloud. For the average person, exposure at any time from Ascension Day should be limited to half an hour on any area of skin for the first day. Provided no painful reaction results, exposure time can be doubled each day, or every other day, for three to six days, depending on results. One should aim at a skin flushed but not painful at the end of the day, gradually darkening from day to day. Too much exposure will make the skin tender, painful, or even blistered, and shade must be sought until the reaction settles, calamine lotion or calamine cream or cold tea being applied every hour or two and *aspirins* or *paracetamol* tablets in the usual doses. Most people find the use of proprietary suntan oils or creams a help in properly regulated sun-bathing, and some are enthusiastic about tablets obtainable from pharmacists, but the expert's tools are patience and a parasol.

There is a wide variation in susceptibility to sunburn and one soon learns one's limitations. Some special cases may be mentioned:

1 Some drugs used for the treatment of depression and some antibiotic and sulphonamide drugs can increase the risk of sunburn. The latter are most likely to be used for the long-term treatment of urinary infection, such as repeated attacks of *cystitis* and *pyelitis*.
2 Exposure to sun while suffering from a 'cold sore' (see *Herpes simplex*) can cause a reaction of the skin.
3 A few people are so sensitive to sunshine that they need special protective creams. These are different from the 'suntan' creams and oils and are ordered by the doctor or skin specialist.
4 Sufferers from pulmonary *tuberculosis* should not sunbathe without medical advice.

Sunstroke. The old name for the conditions now known as heat stroke and heat exhaustion. Heat stroke is almost unknown in temperate climates. It is a dangerous illness occurring in very hot wet climates, usually in someone already ill with, eg, malaria or dysentery. Heat exhaustion may be met with if moist thundery air complicates a heat wave, or if such conditions are simulated at work. In these circumstances anyone doing heavy work will lose so much salt in his sweat that his body runs short of it, and the patient collapses with nausea, faintness, and a cold moist skin.

The treatment is to rest the patient in a cool place and give frequent drinks of water containing 600 mg (about the same bulk as that of two *aspirin* tablets) of common salt in each pint (500 ml). If the patient does not recover in the course of an hour or so, or if he loses consciousness, the doctor should be called (**U** or **UU**). Do not try to give drink to an unconscious patient.

After an attack, heavy work should not be undertaken for several days, and in any subsequent heat wave the patient should drink salted water as above, a pint every hour or two while doing heavy work.

Note that the effect is not produced by the direct rays of the sun (see *Sunburn*) but by hot damp working conditions.

Swollen Feet and Legs. Can arise from many causes. As these include: gnat bites; flat foot; abdominal tumours; phlebitis — inflamed or clotted veins; certain kinds of heart and kidney trouble; and an inborn tendency to swollen feet, it will be seen that this is not a subject for amateurs, and medical advice should be taken (**C** or **D**). In particular, if swelling is sudden, painful and worse when standing on the leg, it may be due to a clotted vein (see *Thrombosis*) and no attempt should be made to stand or walk on the leg. Rest in or on a bed until the doctor sees it.

Sudden swelling of both legs during pregnancy may be serious. Rest in bed until seen — **D**, or **U** if there is also headache.

Syphilis. One of the *venereal diseases*, spread by sexual intercourse. It is not a good subject for guesswork, and any sore developing in the genital region should be seen by the doctor (**S**), as the earlier diagnosis and treatment, the better the chance of complete cure. Those fearing that they have run a risk of venereal infection should not wait for something to appear, but should report to doctor or *VD centre* as soon as possible.

Teething. The age at which teeth appear and the order of their appearance varies. Usually, two lower front teeth erupt first, between 5 and 10 months, then all four upper front teeth before a year. The other lower front and the first molars 2 months later, and the 'eye teeth' ('canines') before the second birthday. The second molars appear during the third year.

Although many children cut teeth without any trouble, a number become fretful and feverish, and a few have vomiting or loose stools for a few days. These symptoms cease as soon as the tooth is cut, and if they do not, some other cause should be suspected. The side of the face in which the tooth is on the move may be flushed, and the child may be in obvious discomfort, which can often be relieved by *paracetamol* or *aspirin in the careful dosage described under those headings*. Sometimes the extra saliva found in the mouth can cause a cough when it runs back and irritates the throat. Tilting the head end of the cot up a few inches can help this.

A child prone to *eczema, asthma*, or *nettle rash* may have an attack while teething, which clears afterwards.

It should not be assumed that serious illness is caused by uncomplicated teething, and medical advice should never be delayed in that belief. Some children are said to 'cut their teeth with bronchitis'; perhaps because teething temporarily lowers resistance, so that infection gains a hold. The bronchitis needs the doctor's care just as much, whether the child is teething or not (**D**).

The use of a bone or suitable plastic teething ring is a help, if it is too large to be swallowed (tie a tape on it anyway) and is regularly sterilized by boiling for five minutes.

Temperature Taking (see also *Fever*). A useful procedure in the right hands. For purposes of home medicine it is best used during the first half of the day, so that the doctor can be told before his round if a visit is indicated. A temperature of 100 degrees F or more in the morning or at midday may be expected to reach 102 to 104 at night, and everyone will then wish that help had been summoned earlier. A temperature reading, even if below 100 degrees, may be a help to the doctor in deciding if a home visit is necessary, in view of his knowledge of the prevalent illnesses, the patient (and the temperature taker!).

Method: Invest in the best; a stub-ended clinical thermometer with magnifying scale, ie, one whose glass is pear-shaped in section, rather than round. Make sure the end of the mercury is below the arrow which marks 98.6 degrees. If it is not, hold firmly and give one or two shakes, shaking the mercury end away from you. Having been washed in cold water, the stub end is placed under the patient's tongue, and he then holds the thermometer between closed lips, steadying it with his hand if necessary. After five minutes it is removed and held so that the scale is being looked at squarely. Gently rotate the thermometer a few degrees backwards and forwards, when the magnifying wedge on the glass will broaden the appearance of the thread of mercury. Where this broad appearance ends on the scale is the temperature reading. Note that the arrow at 98.6 degrees (new standard, the old was 98.4) marks the upper limit of the normal range of the

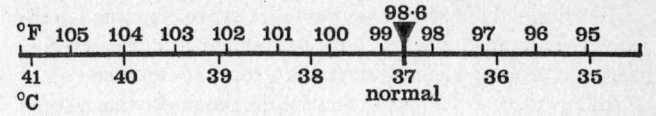

°F	105	104	103	102	101	100	99	98.6 ▼ 98	97	96	95
°C	41	40	39	38		37 normal			36		35

Comparison of Centigrade and Fahrenheit temperatures

temperature. One does not have to score exactly that figure, and readings of two degrees below it are quite common in cold weather. The thermometer is marked in degrees — 98, 99, 100, etc, and the small scale between the degrees is in tenths of a degree. For practical purposes, these are not important. It is important not to confuse 100.4 (100 degrees plus 4 little divisions on the way up to 101) with a hundred *and* four near the top end of the thermometer. If in doubt, do not try to be too clever; simply say 'between 100 and 101'. These are Fahrenheit scale, with which we in the U.K. are still most familiar, but the change to Centigrade, now officially Celsius, is proceeding fast, and a comparative scale is shown. If the patient's teeth are chattering or he has not control of himself, the thermometer is placed in the armpit and kept there for five minutes. In young children, the fold of the groin is a suitable place, holding the thigh gently flexed throughout.

Tennis Elbow (see *Pain in elbow*).

Testicles. The paired male genital organs, hanging in a bag (the *scrotum*) below the penis. They are very sensitive, and even minor injury can produce pain sufficient to cause fainting. Two frequent forms of injury are direct violence, often from falling astride something, and twisting ('torsion') of the organ on its stalk. If continuing pain follows a fall or strain, the patient should have medical attention within a few hours. He may need treatment for *shock* before being moved. Painful swelling unconnected with accident is often due to orchitis, inflammation of the testicle. Most commonly a complication of *mumps*, it can be caused by other infections, and needs medical advice (**V** or **S** according to severity — don't go to Surgery with mumps), as does also any painless swelling discovered in the scrotum (**C**).

Until shortly before birth, the testicles are contained in the lower abdomen, whence they pass down into the scrotum through a canal running over the groin. Sometimes one or both has not reached the scrotum at the time of birth, and does so during the first few years of life. If at the age of four years, a testicle is still 'undescended', the boy should be kept under routine supervision by his doctor, in case active treatment is needed. Sometimes the testicle is not only undescended but 'ectopic' — that is, it has taken a wrong turning and is lying outside the canal. A testicle cannot develop its function as a sperm-forming organ at puberty unless it is in the scrotum, hence the need for treatment well before that time. A young boy's testicles may disappear temporarily back into the canals if the muscles are stimulated. This can well happen if undressing in cold weather for a bath, when it is likely to be noticed, with consequent alarm. It is worth re-examination in more relaxed conditions before taking him to the doctor.

It has recently been suggested that the wearing of tight-fitting underpants may reduce the production of sperm by the testicles. These garments are in such wide use, that any effect would seem to be marginal, but a change to 'boxer shorts' style could be considered if a boy's testicles do not seem to be developing to normal size, or if a man shows a low sperm count when investigated for reduced fertility. An open mind should be kept until more information is available. (See also *Puberty, Scrotum, Rupture.*) See illustration, p. 217.

Tetanus. An often fatal disease, caused by infection of a wound or scratch by bacteria which flourish in soil and horse manure. As treatment is not always successful, protection should be secured by *vaccination*. Regular reinforcements (boosters) are important for agricultural workers and those in contact with horses. Any wound that might be contaminated, e.g. in a road accident, should be seen so that immunity can be brought up to date (S or V).

Thrombosis. The formation of a clot in an artery (taking blood *from* the heart to an organ) or vein (returning blood *to* the heart for re-oxygenating). The danger of an arterial thrombosis is that the part of the organ which the blocked artery supplies will have its supply cut off and will quickly die. If this is in the brain, the result will be a *stroke*, of severity dependent on the position and size of the blocked artery. If in the muscular wall of the heart, a 'coronary' thrombosis will put out of action a section of the wall which will be weakened temporarily or permanently. (See also *Coronary attack*.)

A clot forming in a vein may be visible as an inflamed tender area feeling like a piece of cord under the skin, if the vein is near the surface. If a deep vein in a limb is affected, the limb will swell and the skin may become white and shiny. Before this, if a leg vein is affected, pain will develop in the leg shortly after the patient first stands on it from a lying or sitting position. The first time this test is made should be the last, as the patient *must* then lie or sit with the leg supported completely on soft cushions, and not try to get up until the doctor has seen him (D). The danger of thrombosis of a vein (called thrombophlebitis) is that the clot may be dislodged and swept along into the heart. It will do no harm there, but will be pumped out with the blood going to the lungs for re-oxygenation and will lodge in the lungs, causing a pulmonary embolism — a condition which can be mild or very serious, depending on the size of the clot. A patient suffering from 'phlebitis' who suddenly develops pain in the chest and difficulty in breathing, needs a doctor urgently (UU).

It is very rare for a clot to be dislodged from a surface vein, and the doctor will often be able to advise the patient to remain active. A deep vein thrombosis always needs rest, and usually anti-coagulant treatment given either by injection or tablets.

Thrombophlebitis is a rare complication of using an oral contraceptive, and of prolonged sitting, as when travelling.

Thrush. Common name for infection by a wild yeast causing white patches on the lining of the mouth, usually of a bottle-fed infant. The yeast is a normal inhabitant of the intestine of many people, and can be transferred to the feeding apparatus by a failure in sterilizing technique or toilet hygiene. Diagnosis is best made by the doctor (C), who will order treatment.

Thrush can be troublesome in other ways:

1 By causing a vaginal discharge which can continually re-infect a chronic paronychia (see *Finger, poisoned*) (S). Vaginal thrush is more frequent if one is taking a contraceptive 'pill'. Daily cleansing of the skin with warm water and soap should be the rule.
2 After use of an antibiotic, the yeast may be activated, causing inflammation of mouth or rectum. Usually a minor occurrence, it can occasionally be serious in a frail patient (S or occasionally V).

Tinea (see *Ringworm*).

Toadstool Poisoning. Anyone becoming ill after eating what were thought to be mushrooms needs medical care very urgently (UU). If at all possible, try to find a piece of the toadstool that was eaten (from kitchen waste or left-overs) for identification.

The commonest cause, and the most serious, is Amanita Phalloides, which superficially resembles a field mushroom; there may be a delay of 12 to 15 hours before it produces effects.

Unless you are a mycologist, buy your mushrooms from a shop.

If you don't know what a mycologist is, buy your mushrooms from a shop.

Tongue, Furred, etc. The most important thing about a furred tongue is that it is not usually important. Tongues are naturally furry, as can be seen at any butcher's shop, and the amount varies from person to person, and time to time.

When abnormal furring accompanies disease, the disease will usually have drawn attention to itself long before.

Brown or blackish discoloration occurs, sometimes after taking antibiotics or with iron treatment, sometimes spontaneously. It usually disappears if left alone.

Unusual *smoothness* of the tongue may accompany some deficiency conditions, such as anaemia; and there is a harmless patchy irregularity, well described as geographical tongue, for it suggests a map, and is not a disease at all.

The first sight of the very back of one's tongue in a mirror can be alarming if one does not know that the scattered warty hillocks are a normal feature, usually out of sight 'over the hill'.

Aphthous *ulcers* occur on the tongue, and usually clear up within ten days. Any ulcer or sore which does not disappear in a fortnight should be shown to one's doctor (C).

Tonics. The old-fashioned tonic was a medicine designed to improve the general feeling of the taker, after illness, or during an attack of mild melancholia (*depression*). The active ingredient was usually a vegetable bitter or astringent chemical, and the effect was to stimulate the lining of the stomach, in turn increasing the 'tone' of its muscular wall. It seems that one feels better when one's stomach muscle is reasonably active and less so, even positively poorly, when it is not. Often, a mild sedative was included in these mixtures, which, of course, could have no tonic effect, and its purpose was to relax the nervous tension which was contributing to the patient's trouble. (The two properties account for the benefit which many feel after drinking a glass of beer, which has also a mild laxative effect.) The fact that a patient who asks for a tonic is probably suffering from depression or psychological ('nervous') tension, has led to its disparagement in more sophisticated circles, it being thought that attention would be better directed to the psychological cause. In the writer's view, it is reasonable to take a dose of a vegetable bitter (alkaline gentian mixture, two 5 ml spoonfuls before meals in a little water) for a week or so after an acute illness, or when faced with a *mild* bout of depression. It would be useless in a depression of any severity, and should not be allowed to delay medical treatment in such a case (see *Depression*).

A glass of vermouth (French or Italian) before a meal could take the place of the gentian mixture, if preferred; many connoisseurs recommend a glass of stout drunk during the midday meal.

Tonsillitis. See general statement under *Adenoids* and *Tonsils*. An attack of tonsillitis results when inhaled bacteria settle in the throat and are engaged by the body's defences, using the tonsils as a battlefield. Onset is sudden, with feeling of acute illness, rising temperature and pain in the throat, increasing after the first few hours. The tonsils at the back of the throat are seen to be red, swollen, and to have several white or yellow spots. The lymph nodes (*glands*) under the angles of the jaw are swollen and tender, and it hurts to swallow. The temperature remains high for two or three nights, then falls, and the patient improves more or less steadily. The need for medical help depends on the severity of the infection (**D** or **V**). Mild cases will manage on *aspirin* or *paracetamol* tablets, three or four times in 24 hours, and copious drinks. Others may need antibiotic treatment. Children, young adults and anyone who has in the past had either *rheumatic fever* or *nephritis* should always have medical help at the onset of tonsillitis.

In tonsillitis caused by a particular type of streptococcus, the poison absorbed from the system may give rise to a rash over most of the body on the second or third day. This is a toxic rash, and if severe, it constitutes a case of *Scarlet fever* (**D** or **V**).

Toothache. Mild toothache may be relieved by *aspirin* or *paracetamol* tablets and frequent mouth washes of warm *isotonic saline*; raising the head end of the bed 5–7 inches helps. A badly diseased tooth may be eased temporarily by swilling with a little neat brandy or whisky (but do not combine aspirin and alcohol). None of these will help an abscess much, and the sooner the dentist can deal with the tooth the better. As he may need to give a general anaesthetic ('gas'), no food or drink should be taken within four hours of the appointment, otherwise the extraction may have to be postponed. Even the mildest toothache indicates that a dental appointment should be made.

Travel. The Department of Health and Social Security publishes advice to travellers abroad in a booklet called *Health Protection*, free from Alexander Fleming House, Elephant and Castle, London SE1 6BY. Send stamped addressed envelope, preferably eight weeks before travelling, to allow time for vaccinations.

Travel Sickness. A feeling of general illness with nausea and vomiting experienced by many people when in a moving car, boat, or aircraft. It is made much worse by anxiety, emotional disturbance, and loss of confidence, bred of previous attacks. It is caused by stimulation of the vomiting reflex of the brain and the autonomic nervous network of the body, and may be related to receipt by the brain of conflicting messages about what is happening. Thus, if the victim is sitting in the back of a car, or cabin of a boat, his eyes will inform his brain that his surroundings (coachwork or cabin furniture) are still, in relation to himself, while his balancing organs (see in *Vertigo*) will tell him that his head is moving up and down, or in other directions. Prevention is by:

1 Reducing the sensory contradictions mentioned above. If one stands at the rail of a boat, looking outwards, one will feel that one is going up and down and confirm it by sight of the sea. Lying flat in the cabin with the eyes shut allows the sensation of rising and falling felt with one's back to be confirmed by the balancing organs. Most people are more confident with feet lying towards the bows, than otherwise. In a car, up and down movement is less in the front seats than the back, and is more easily related to the forward view of the road. If making use of a reclining seat, the eyes should be kept closed. In aircraft, if the seat cannot be made fully reclining, the best position is

crouched forward with head well down, holding the paper bag between the knees, and with the eyes closed.
2 Reducing the effect of the disturbance of the nervous system by taking hyoscine, Avomine, Marzine or Dramamine, or such other treatment as the doctor may order, at least an hour before the journey. Hyoscine is obtainable as 'Kwells' and this and other remedies should be used according to the makers' recommendation.

Note: All these can affect driving ability adversely.

Both in the long-and short-term, one gets used to travelling without sickness. On a short sea voyage or 'plane trip, the precautions described should be taken. On a long voyage, most people can confidently expect to become free in a day or two, with the possible exception of a mild queasiness on first rising, dispelled by going on deck. Stormy conditions must be met by the measures outlined above.

Children, if managed sensibly, grow out of the tendency. The driver should drive slowly enough to avoid roll on corners, avoid rapid changes of speed, ensure a good current of air through the car, and make frequent stops to stroll for a few minutes, without mentioning the possibility of sickness. A watch is kept for any passenger who drops out of the conversation, and a halt made without comment. A child who announces that he is always sick in cars may be told before starting that people are not sick in this car.

Tuberculosis. Infection of any part of the body by a particular germ, the tubercle bacillus. The result differs from almost all other infective processes in lasting for years rather than days or weeks. Any part of the body can be affected, but since the elimination of tuberculosis from dairy herds, infection of joints, neck 'glands', and abdominal organs has become rare, and it is assumed that these usually arose from infected milk. Tuberculosis of the lungs ('pulmonary tuberculosis'), spread by the cough of infected patients, is still a wasteful disease, though its main onslaught has now shifted to the higher age-groups, away from the adolescents and young adults who were its chief victims 25 years ago. This has been achieved by a combination of measures, including the testing of older schoolchildren by the Mantoux test, which shows whether the child has already suffered tuberculous infection, as many have, particularly town dwellers. X-ray of the lungs of the 'positive reactors' shows whether they have successfully overcome the chance infection and derived resistance to further infection thereby, or whether they are at that time in the grip of a primary infection, which has not yet been overcome. If the latter, they will be kept under observation, perhaps with some limitation of activity, and treatment, until the infection is successfully overcome. Those who react negatively to the Mantoux test — that is, have never experienced any tuberculous infection — are assumed to be at risk of infection, and are advised to undergo immunization by means of a single *vaccination* with BCG vaccine. This produces a small lump or sore at the site of the injection in the arm which may last for some weeks or even months, allowing immunity to develop, so that subsequent Mantoux tests show them as 'positive'. The early recognition of cases of lung tuberculosis by mass X-ray and by family doctors investigating stubborn *coughs*, has resulted in less chance infection from patients, and the wonderful improvements in chemical treatment of the disease have greatly reduced the time before the average case is able to return to work — *provided the case is taken early*.

Always report to the doctor:

1 Coughing of blood or bloodstained phlegm.
2 A cough lasting more than two or three weeks.
3 Loss of weight.

Typhoid Fever (Enteric Fever). A severe infection of the intestines which can take several forms in the early stages, and is usually diagnosed by means of laboratory tests. There is a milder form, paratyphoid. Uncommon in this country, but the risk of infection, except in Northern Europe and North America, is sufficient to make *vaccination* advisable before travelling.

Outbreaks of typhoid in Great Britain usually happen when

food or water is contaminated by someone who unknowingly carries the infection without being ill. As the germs are excreted from the bowel or bladder, most outbreaks should be prevented by washing the hands after using the lavatory, and before preparing or eating food. (See also *Carrier*.)

U and I. The U and I Club provides advice to people troubled by repeated urinary infection, or incontinence. Send stamped addressed envelope for particulars to 9E Compton Road, London N1.

Ulcer. A breach in one of the surfaces of the body, external or internal. An ulcer on the outside of the body results if an area of skin is removed full-thickness by wound or burn, or is deprived of conditions necessary for its survival, as by the reduction of its blood supply. Whatever the cause, the appearance is of a hole in the skin through which the deeper tissues appear, sometimes covered with pus, caused by bacteria spreading themselves on exposed flesh. Occasionally a tumour formed below the skin burrows outwards, cutting off the overlying skin's blood supply, and is then said to 'ulcerate' through the skin. Common sites for an ulcer are the lower leg or foot, where the circulation of the skin is already rather poor and where *varicose veins* or *diabetes* can depress conditions below the level at which healing takes place, so that a minor knock or scratch can lead to breakdown of the skin.

Serious internal ulcers are *gastric* and *duodenal*; in these the breach is in the lining of the stomach or the duodenal tube leading from it. A common mild ulcer is the aphthous type, found in the mouth, varying in size from one-sixteenth of an inch to one-third of an inch. The cause of these is not known and they usually heal themselves in five to ten days — if not, doctor's advice should be taken (C). Their main effect is the constant pain they cause; it is worth taking courage and rubbing them with a sludge made from an aspirin tablet and one or two drops of water. Done once or twice a day, this usually relieves pain. Aphthous ulcers apart, any others are subjects for medical diagnosis and treatment — even then, some take long enough to heal (C).

Unconsciousness (see also *Electric shock*). A patient is found lying in bed or fallen, apparently asleep, and cannot be wakened. Make sure there is no immediate danger, eg, from mechanical or electrical causes. Ascertain that breathing is free and not obstructed by clotted blood, vomit, displaced dentures, etc. Free any obstruction found. If not breathing, proceed as in *Artificial respiration*.

Once breathing is satisfactory, unless there is reason to suspect spine or neck injury, turn the patient into the 'semi-prone' position illustrated, drawing up the free leg and arm as stabilizers, the face to the side and a little downward. If help is at hand, try to turn body in one piece — head, shoulder, and

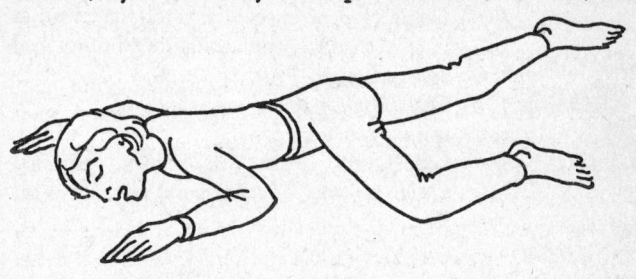

The position in which an unconscious breathing person should be placed

hip at the same time — to avoid twisting the spine (see *Injuries*).

Next carefully and gently examine for any *bleeding*, and if any is found, stop it. A doctor, ambulance, or first aid worker is urgently needed (UU) and unless the patient is in a position of imminent danger (fire or gas — see *Gas or Fume* poisoning) the next priority is to send for, or secure, such help. That done, consider the common causes of unconsciousness and the clues which knowledge, observation, or inquiry can give to them:

- **If a patient is not within the scope of home care, or worsens in spite of it, or if there is any uncertainty, a doctor should be consulted.**

248 Urine

Brain Injury Signs of violence.
(See *Concussion*) Wound of skull.
Traces of blood at site of fall.
Patient at foot of stairs, history of recent head injury, etc.

Stroke History of treatment for high blood pressure.
History of previous strokes or heart disease.

Diabetes Coma of quick onset due to too little sugar in system. Known diabetic may have lost a meal through vomiting or omitted to eat it due to *gastritis*.
Coma of slow onset due to too little insulin in system. Deep breathing (well described as 'air hunger')

Poisoning Overdose of drugs — traces of package, spilled tablets, etc.
Gas, fumes — see *Gas or Fume poisoning*.
Other poisons — containers, acid burns on skin.

Any conclusion you can draw and pass on will save time when treatment is started.

Further action is limited to preventing the patient from losing body heat, by wrapping in blankets, particularly protecting feet and hands. The patient should be moved as little as possible until help arrives. An injured patient should only be moved if in danger from his surroundings (see *Injuries*), and if there is any suspicion of violence the surroundings should not be disturbed, except where essential to wrap the patient. No additional heat is needed, and no attempt should be made to give any food or drink.

Drowning is considered under its own heading.

Consult the entry *Death* for distinction between coma and death.

Urine. The kidneys extract waste and surplus matter from the circulation, filter and concentrate them, and pass the resulting fluid down to the bladder for storage and eventual excretion

If these products were harmless, there would be no need to get rid of them, and any action which prolongs their contact with the body can be expected to do more harm than good. Thus, nappies should be changed when wet, and waterproof knickers should be regarded as a short-term social convenience when travelling or visiting, and not as a permanent item of clothing.

Frequent or excessive urination needs investigation. It may be frequent because infection irritates and stimulates the bladder (*cystitis, pyelitis*), excessive because more is being produced, as in *diabetes* and some forms of *nephritis*, or following excessive intake of fluid. The frequent, often painful, passage of small quantities, with a scalding feeling after the passage, is suggestive of *cystitis*.

Reduction in the amount of urine passed happens naturally and conveniently at night, when the kidneys produce a reduced volume of more concentrated urine. In chronic *nephritis*, the power of concentration may be reduced, so that more of a dilute urine needs passing during the night. Night rising, general frequency, and incomplete emptying can all be caused by pressure on the male bladder from an enlarged *prostate gland*. Reduced bladder control in women is often due to stretching of the pelvic tissues (see *Prolapse*). Marked reduction in the amount of urine passed, particularly by a child a week or two after a sore throat, suggests acute *nephritis*. It requires early medical advice (D). Inability to pass water, more common in males, can be caused by obstruction to the bladder outflow and as soon as the bladder becomes uncomfortable, the patient should get himself to doctor or hospital (see also *Prostate*).

The colour of urine when passed varies from that of water to deep yellow. It may be coloured pink after eating beetroot, and this may be mistaken for *bleeding*. A *specimen* should be taken to the doctor (S) if there is any doubt. A very dark, sometimes brown, urine may be the first warning of an attack of *jaundice*. (See also *Kidney disease, Prostate, Specimen of urine*.)

Vaccination. The production of resistance to an infectious disease by stimulating the development of antibodies in the system. In International Sanitary Regulations, the term applies to any disease, though in this country 'vaccination' is usually understood to mean protection against *smallpox*, other diseases being covered by the terms 'immunization' and 'inoculation'.

For residents in the United Kingdom, the latest recommendations are as follows; they may be carried out in health centre clinics or by the general practitioner.

During the first year of life. First, second and third doses of diphtheria and tetanus vaccine with or without whooping cough vaccine (see p. 259), together with three doses of oral polio vaccine. It is now recommended that the first dose be given at the age of three months.

During the second year of life. Measles vaccine.

Start of school or nursery. Not earlier than three years after first year course, reinforcement ('booster') doses of diphtheria and tetanus and oral polio vaccines.

Between 11 and 13 years. BCG vaccination against *tuberculosis* and, for girls only, German measles (rubella) vaccination. The latter is also available, after preliminary tests, to women of child-bearing age (see p. 126).

School-leaving (before employment or further education). Reinforcement doses of polio and tetanus.

Adults. Polio vaccination if not already vaccinated, and if going to places where poliomyelitis occurs; or as a precaution against infection from a child who is being given oral vaccine.

Tetanus vaccination for previously unvaccinated adults. Needs reinforcement at about five-year intervals. See *Tetanus*. A record card should be carried showing the injection dates.

German measles (rubella). (See p. 126.)

Influenza. A single injection of vaccine usually increases resistance to infection for several months. People with heart, or bronchial trouble should consult their doctor about this in the autumn.

Common cold. No effective vaccine exists. 'Anti-catarrh' vaccines are sometimes used as a partial protection against complications of the common cold, and those in whom they are successful have great confidence in them.

Overseas travellers. Up-to-date information may be

obtained from 'Health Protection', (see *Travel*), or from the Embassy or High Commission of the country concerned. Smallpox vaccination may be needed; it is no longer required in the United Kingdom, (see *Smallpox*).

Typhoid and paratyphoid vaccination (TAB). This is advisable before travelling beyond northern Europe or North America. Two injections at intervals of two to four weeks (the longer interval gives better protection). Each may produce a feverish reaction during the following 24 hours, and the injection should be arranged so that the patient can rest if necessary. Physical exertion and alcohol should be avoided for 24 hours after each injection. Feverishness responds to *aspirin* or *paracetamol* tablets, and *hot packs* will ease a sore arm.

Cholera. An effective vaccine is available, often combined with TAB for immunization of those travelling abroad, as cholera is now established in parts of Europe. An International Certificate as for smallpox is required. When given alone, the vaccine rarely produces any reaction; if combined with TAB vaccine the reaction to the typhoid part may be expected.

Yellow fever. This is obtainable only in special centres for those proceeding to yellow fever areas. Particulars are usually given with travelling instructions. An International Certificate is required.

Hepatitis. Ask your doctor about possible temporary protection.

Notes. Before vaccination against *smallpox*, the doctor should be told if the patient has any tendency to *eczema* or *nettlerash*, or if anyone in the household is so affected. Anyone with an active vaccination sore, and soiled dressings from it, should be kept well away from anyone suffering from eczema.

After smallpox vaccination usually little happens for five or six days. Then a sore red lump forms with surrounding reddening of the skin. The lump becomes a blister, then a scab forms and healing goes on under that. Finally, the scab falls off leaving a clean scar of varying size and appearance. If vaccination has been done before the reaction may be of less extent and may start sooner. Little treatment is needed for the average vaccination sore, beyond keeping it dry and covered preferably with a pad of gauze, to permit ventilation, and held in position by a cross of narrow adhesive plaster. It should be remembered that the discharge can cause further sores if carried by the dressing or fingers; eyes can become infected in this way. Discarded dressings should be burned and hands washed. Pain, and later, itching, usually respond to *aspirin*. If the skin involvement around the sore is more than 5 to 7.5 cm (2 to 3 inches) across, or if there is much swelling, the doctor should see it (S). Occasionally, symptoms of general illness occur when the reaction is at its height, and for these the doctor should be called (V). If travelling abroad, an International Vaccination Certificate may be needed (obtainable from a travel agency, and doctors usually have a supply). The certificate has to be completed by the doctor who carries out the vaccination.

Before vaccination against whooping cough, or with 'triple' vaccine, the doctor should be told if there is a family history of fits or convulsions, or if any of the conditions described under whooping cough vaccination (p. 30) are present.

Triple vaccine i.e. diphtheria, tetanus and whooping cough, and certain other vaccines, should not be used if poliomyelitis is prevalent, or if the patient contemplates going to a poliomyelitis area during the following few weeks.

For a few weeks after oral poliomyelitis vaccination, the patient may excrete vaccine from his bowel, and this has occasionally caused poliomyelitis in close contacts not already vaccinated. One should prevent contact of a recently vaccinated baby with a child who has not been vaccinated, and the obvious hygienic precautions should be taken in dealing with soiled napkins etc. Close contacts can be given oral vaccine at the same time as the child, if they are not already protected.

Varicocele (see *Scrotum*).

Varicose Veins. Enlarged and tortuous veins seen under the skin of the legs. Any but the mildest will need treatment or support (C). If injured, a vein may bleed alarmingly, but the bleeding stops when the patient lies down with his leg raised in the air. A clean pad (see *dressings*) is pressed firmly on the bleeding point for about ten minutes, then bound on (firmly but not tightly), and the leg lowered to the couch or bed. If bleeding recommences, the leg is raised and pressure applied again, through the dressing. The leg should be kept level overnight and the doctor asked to see it the next day (S or D), or before, if bleeding re-starts.

Vasectomy. A minor operation to produce *permanent* male sterility as a contraceptive measure. Because it is permanent, it should only be undertaken after full consideration by all concerned. The operation is done under local anaesthetic as an out-patient, or under a short general anaesthetic with an overnight stay. The result cannot be relied on until two negative sperm tests, several months after operation.

Venereal Disease (VD). A group of diseases almost wholly spread by sexual intercourse; now officially included in the Sexually Transmitted Diseases. The most serious are *gonorrhoea* and *syphilis*. If not fully and completely treated, these diseases can cripple, kill, or blind, many years after the original infection. Usually the first sign of syphilis is a sore at the point of genital contact, some two to four weeks later. (It will be understood that in the female, this may not be visible externally.) The signs of gonorrhoea are described under that heading. In the course of some weeks, even if untreated, the signs of both diseases will diminish. *The chances of cure are doing the same.* Anyone developing pain, discharge of pus, sore or swelling in or around the genital parts within six weeks of intercourse should visit a doctor (S) or a *VD centre* without delay; and since infection can occur without giving rise to early symptoms, it is best that anyone who has made a casual and unprotected sexual contact should present himself similarly.

Anyone who is found to have a venereal infection should make every effort to persuade his or her contact and any subsequent contacts of either, to be examined. This embarrassing duty, if properly performed, can save endless misery. Infection in women may be unnoticed in its early stages, though the later effects can be more serious than for men; and the increased spread of VD may be partly due to the popularity of the 'pill', through which the considerable protection given by wearing a sheath has been lost.

Anyone approaching marriage, who has been promiscuous, should present him/herself for examination and testing to exclude the possibility of infecting the marriage partner.

'Non-specific urethritis' is now very prevalent. Its symptoms resemble those of *gonorrhoea* and most cases respond well to a full course of treatment.

Almost all venereal disease can be cured if treated early.

Further Reading
Sex and V.D. by Derek Llewellyn-Jones (Faber and Faber).

VD Centre. In all large towns there are centres for the diagnosis and treatment of *venereal diseases*, attendance at which does not need any introduction by the patient's doctor, and where treatment is confidential. Times for attendance are usually displayed in public lavatories and in the public notices of local newspapers. Failing these, an inquiry by telephone or at the inquiry desk of the nearest general hospital for the times of the 'Special Men's/Women's Clinic' will usually produce information without embarrassment.

Verruca (see *Warts*).

Vertigo. An attack of giddiness, sometimes violent, with a feeling that the patient is rotating or falling. There are numerous causes, and one of the commonest is a 'catarrhal' infection causing inflammation of one of the two balancing organs (minute mechanisms placed deep in the sides of the skull, close to the hearing organs) which keep the brain informed of the position of each side of the head in space. When one of these misbehaves, the brain receives conflicting messages from the two sides, which it interprets as meaning that one side of the head and body is spinning round the other. Messages are sent to the muscles on one side to correct the supposed spin, and to the eyes to swivel very fast to keep pace with it. The body is not twisting, of course, and the force of the unneeded correction may be enough to throw the patient out of bed, or if walking, to fall sideways.

All this results in a stimulation of the vomiting centre of the brain, whose effects are then added to the patient's misery. *Treatment:* A first attack is very frightening, and every effort must be made to persuade the patient to lie on his back with the hollow of the neck supported on a *butterfly pillow*. In this position, activity of the balancing organs is kept at a minimum, but any attempt to turn the head may produce an attack. A guarded *hot water bottle* is put to the soles of the feet and the doctor is asked to call (**U** or **D**).

It may be that Avomine or Dramamine tablets for *travel* or *pregnancy* sickness are available. If so, crush half one to a powder and give mixed in a teaspoon with milk or milk and water. After 20 minutes, give the other half. If the patient can retain these for an hour, they will begin to ease the severity of the attack.

This treatment can be adopted for vertigo due to any cause, such as that arising when an older person over-stretches the neck in the course of sleep, or by looking upwards, kinking the blood vessels which supply the balancing system.

Another cause of vertigo is Ménière's disease, in which attacks are associated with deafness and/or ringing in the ears. Sufferers are usually aware of their disability, and already have treatment for it, but a first attack should be managed in the way described above.

Virus. The term usually means 'filter-passing virus' — a large group of minute organisms many times smaller than ordinary bacteria. (See *Germs*.)

Vitamins. Substances present in minute amounts in natural food, which are needed for the maintenance of health. The ordinary mixed diet in the United Kingdom has sufficient vitamins, and ill-health from vitamin deficiency is believed to be rare. It can happen when older people living alone become uninterested in buying and preparing food, and it is as well when visiting them to try to form an idea of the state of their larder. If they seem to be living mainly on bread or chips, and fruit, vegetables or dairy foods are not to be seen, they may need help, either by the more regular visit of a friend or relative; perhaps by being put in touch with the Meals on Wheels Service, or through the Health Visitor. Until children are weaned on to a mixed diet, their intake of vitamins may be inadequate, and they are usually given vitamin preparations in the form of drops or liquid. As dried milk may contain added vitamins, there is a danger of giving more than a safe intake of vitamin D if the quantities advised by the clinic, health visitor or doctor are exceeded.

A difficult older child who forms an aversion to food may go short of vitamins if the reduced or limited intake lasts several weeks. The problem is not usually an acute one, and the doctor will advise about it.

Although it is not known that giving additional quantities of vitamins to someone whose intake is already sufficient has any good effect, many people do take vitamin concentrates and some of them believe that they are fitter, and resist infection better, while doing so. There is no scientific confirmation of this, but perhaps an open mind should be kept.

It is possible that low vitamin intake before and after conception may play a part in the production of congenital deformities.

Vomiting. Return of food, etc, from the stomach into the mouth. Causes:

1 Infected food in the stomach (food poisoning); some chemical poisons.
2 Normal food which an inflamed stomach cannot retain (acute *gastritis*).
3 Excessive intake of food and/or drink causing inflammation of stomach (carelessness).
4 Back-pressure from obstruction in the intestines.
5 Messages reaching the stomach from the brain or nervous system:
   (a) *Vertigo;*
   (b) *Travel sickness;*

(c) *Migraine;*
(d) Nauseating sight or sound;
(e) Acute pain as from twisted knee, etc;
(f) Infection or damage to brain;
(g) As a complication of some forms of medical treatment.

Treatment: **1** and **2** may be indistinguishable unless others who have eaten infected food are also affected. The treatment is that of acute gastritis (see *Gastroenteritis*). Some of the vomit from the early stages should be saved in a cleansed (preferably scalded) covered container, in case laboratory examination becomes necessary. In some cases of food poisoning, the patient becomes prostrated and is obviously seriously ill. A doctor should be called (**U**).

3 Half a 5 ml spoonful of bicarbonate of soda in a little water when the situation is first recognized. Sips of milk and water mixture (50–50) between bouts of vomiting.

4 Much less common. May be suspected if vomiting persists in a patient who has passed neither motion nor wind from the bowel for several days, or who has a *rupture* (hernia) which does not replace itself. Sometimes the condition degenerates in the course of a few hours, the vomit becomes brown and smells foul. Call a doctor (**U**).

5 (*a, b, c*) See under their separate headings.

(*d, e*) Will subside without treatment. If practicable, patient should lie down or sit with head on knees for some minutes.

(*f*) Patient is obviously ill, even unconscious (**U** or **UU**).

(*g*) Notify whoever ordered the treatment. Meanwhile, treat as **1** and **2**.

An unconscious or semi-conscious patient is in danger of inhaling vomit. Treat as described under *Unconsciousness*. (A child should be held tilted with head lower than feet and face downward.)

Warts. These enigmatic growths, usually on the fingers, are caused by an infectious *virus*, and can spread by contact. The enigma lies in the fact that in some people, some warts can be made to disappear by suggestion — that is, by giving strong assurance to the patient that the warts will go, but giving no effective treatment to the warts themselves. Some people are reputed to be particularly successful at 'charming' warts. A method sometimes used and worth trying in younger children is to suggest to them that they sell the warts to someone, who offers them, say 5p for them. The money is passed over on the understanding that when the warts are found to have gone they have become the property of the purchaser. Many of the country remedies for warts are probably effective by suggestion. There are various medical measures of treatment, and some are more successful than others. Occasionally it is found that when several treatments have failed and been abandoned, a heavy crop of warts disappears overnight. Warts on the thick non-hairy skin of soles and palms are called verrucas. They are not raised, but grow into the thickness of the skin. They are often spread in swimming baths and school changing rooms, and like other warts occasionally die without treatment. Few sufferers are prepared to wait for this if the verruca is on the weight-bearing area of the foot, and the doctor should be consulted (C).

Wax in Ears (see *Deafness*).

Whitlow (see *Finger, poisoned*).

Whooping Cough (Pertussis). In a typical case, after a cough has lasted ten days or so, the characteristic whoop develops. This whoop is a drawing *intake* of breath after a spasm of coughing, in the course of which the patient may become red or purple in the face. It is not part of the noise of the cough — the so-called 'croupy cough' in which a hoarse wheezy sound forms part of the cough is nothing to do with whooping cough (see under *Cough*). The spasms, sometimes associated with vomiting, persist for some two weeks, then gradually abate. The doctor should be asked to see the child (V) when the whoop first appears, or before, if the patient's condition requires it.

The spasms of whooping cough, if severe, can be alarming. In young children, it is best to hold them with head and mouth downwards at the end of a spasm or during vomiting, so that when they take the eventual gasp of breath they do not inhale any vomit or saliva from the mouth. Anyone who has experienced an attack will wish to gain the protection of immunization (see *Vaccination*) for young children. It may not prevent an attack, but an attack in an immunized patient is usually mild — so much so, that diagnosis may be difficult. (See p. 250).

Alarm may be caused by the tendency for simple coughs to follow the whooping cough pattern, with spasm and even whoops, for the first year or two after a known attack of whooping cough. These are not due to re-infection, and will not spread whooping cough.

Incubation Period: 7–14 days.

Quarantine: Of patient, 28 days from the beginning of the 'characteristic cough'.

Of contacts, 21 days from the start of the illness.

'Wind'. The term covers the belching of air upwards and the passing of gas downwards. Belching results when excessive air is introduced into the stomach. This can happen as a neurotic habit, or deliberately to relieve discomfort in the stomach. If the latter, the cause of the discomfort must be sought by the doctor (C). Much more frequently, the air is swallowed when food is swallowed jerkily. This may happen occasionally at a hurried meal, or regularly because the eater is in a state of nervous and muscular tension while eating. As a result, food is thrown backwards by the tongue and gulped down with a bubble of air, instead of being *squeezed* back into the gullet by a smooth swallowing movement. Relief will be found in the cultivation of *relaxation* and the setting aside of sufficient time for the leisured consumption of the meal. Note that almost without exception, what is belched is air, not gas. The only gas likely to be belched is carbon dioxide released from a fizzy drink.

Flatulence, on the other hand, is caused by gas released in the lower bowel by the processes of digestive fermentation. It is natural for some to be passed, but some people are luckier than others, presumably owing to differing constitution. Certain foods — notoriously beans — may be found to increase flatulence, and some possessors of a 'greedy colon', which extracts excessive quantities of water from the contents of the lower intestine, also suffer. They are often helped by the practice of regular water drinking. (See *Aperients*.)

Flatulence may increase for a few weeks after starting a bran or other high-residue diet, but a persistent increase should lead a patient to consult his doctor, as should also inability to pass any (C). 'Wind' in infants is discussed in the chapter *Newborn*.

Worms. Several kinds of worm-shaped animals can make their homes in the human intestine. They may become apparent when their anchorage fails and they are passed by a motion of the bowel. In the nature of things, this will be noticed more often when a child is the host, and by far the commonest infestation is by thread worms. Usually, a child of school age who has noticed some itching around the anus, particularly at night, is found to have passed a motion in which a number, sometimes a great number, of thread worms are seen. They resemble short lengths (about half an inch) of chopped linen thread, dirty white in colour.

In the subsequent alarm, two things should be remembered. There is little or no effect on the general health, though the victim may be made short-tempered by itching, and by the remarks of such of her family as are unaware of the second point. This is that the infestation is frequently shared by many or all of the members of a household. The next step is to make an inspection of each one's motion. In some, there may be only a few worms, or none. The patient, and the result of these investigations, are now taken to the doctor (C), who may advise treatment for the patient alone, or for the whole family if necessary. Treatment is painless and harmless.

Prevention depends on a knowledge of the life cycle of the worm. The victim first swallows unaware some of the microscopical eggs of the worm which have been transferred to his fingers from those of someone already infested. Once inside, the eggs hatch into worms, which then inhabit the patient's lower bowel, coming out at night to deposit their eggs in the skin around the anus. The scratching of this skin lodges eggs under the finger nails which are then transferred to the mouth, or to somebody else's fingers, and the process repeats itself. The finger nails should be trimmed short and a *soft* nailbrush used each morning, and before feeding. The doctor may order internal treatment, and the application at bedtime of ammoniated mercury ointment to the skin around the anus to kill the worms as they emerge.

Far rarer is an infestation with round or tape worms. Proof of these is from the appearance in the motion of (usually) a single worm resembling an earth worm, or several flattened translucent squares or oblongs quarter to half inch long. Either should if possible be rescued and taken to the doctor (C). Failing that, about a teaspoonful of the motion including any gelatinous part, should be taken in a securely closed container.

Dogs and Cats. It is believed that more than one in three of these pets may be infested with their own type of worm, whose minute eggs are passed from the bowel and are easily transferred to the fingers of those handling the animals. If they are subsequently swallowed, the hatched worms bore their way through the tissues of the human host and form themselves into cysts. If these form in the eye or brain, the results can be very serious, and it is important to take veterinary advice *before* introducing a puppy or kitten into a family, to ensure de-worming. Obviously, children should be taught to wash immediately after handling animals, and a child passing through a phase of finger sucking or nail biting should not handle a dog or cat. (See *Animals, domestic.*)

Wounds (see also *Abrasions, Bleeding, Cuts, Dressings, First Aid, Injuries*). The amount of first aid needed for a small or moderate wound depends on how soon it is to come under medical care. If this is within an hour or so, and provided the skin round the wound is not contaminated with loose earth or obviously infected matter, stop the *bleeding*, apply as clean a *dressing* as possible, and take, or send, to a hospital or doctor under such supervision as seems necessary.

If a foreign body is protruding from the wound, arrange the

dressing round it, and try to stabilize it with padding so that it doesn't move in transit.

If several hours must elapse before medical care, the skin round the wound should be cleaned before applying the dressing. Protect the wound with a small clean dressing, leaving as much of the surrounding skin uncovered as possible. Use clean swabs of gauze, lint or cotton wool, sterilized if possible, moistened with 1 per cent Cetrimide in water, discarding them as they become soiled. Work outwards from the edge of the wound and let no drips run into it.

A puncture wound may seem small on the surface, but can disguise a deep injury. All puncture wounds of head, face, eye, chest, abdomen, or near a joint should have medical attention the same day.

Wricked Neck (see *Spondylosis*).

X-rays. Rays which pass through living tissues to a varying extent according to the sort of tissues they encounter. On emerging from the body, they will therefore produce on a photographic film a shadowgraph of the body structures they have passed through. In this, the various layers through which they have passed will be superimposed, and it can be understood that expert interpretation of the film is needed. The idea that an X-ray gives a 'picture' of the internal organs, as though an inspection cover had been removed, is far from the truth.

The development of mass X-rays, using miniature films, has greatly helped in the early recognition and treatment of lung disease, and everyone over forty is advised to attend for this once a year. It is not always possible to judge whether an unusual shadow on a miniature film is of importance, and anyone whose film is in any way abnormal is usually asked to attend a chest clinic so that a full-sized film can be taken and interpreted. The mass X-ray is one of the most important *screening* tests, but it is not suitable for use on adolescents and pregnant mothers.

X-rays of a much more powerful type are used for the treatment of certain diseases. These are quite different in their purpose and effects from those used for taking X-ray films.

- **If a patient is not within the scope of home care, or worsens in spite of it, or if there is any uncertainty, a doctor should be consulted.**

Appendix

One way to know about a disease is to have it; and since H. G. Wells founded the British Diabetic Association in 1934, many other Societies and Associations have been formed to pool the information possessed by sufferers, and to advance their welfare. This list is not complete, and new organizations are being formed all the time. Up-to-date information about particular diseases should be available from Social Workers in Hospitals, or from Local Social Services Departments. If writing direct to an Association, always send a stamped addressed envelope for their reply. Many bodies will refer enquirers to local organizations or groups.

Age Concern, 60 Pitcairn Rd, Mitcham, Surrey CR4 3LL

Alcoholics Anonymous — see alphabetical section.

Alcoholism, National Council on — see Alcoholism.

Arthritis & Rheumatism Council for Research in Great Britain and the Commonwealth, 8/10 Charing Cross Road, London WC2H 0HN

British Diabetic Association, 10 Queen Anne Street, London W1M 0BD

British Dyslexia Association, 18 The Circus, Bath BA1 2ET

British Epilepsy Association, Crowthorne House, Bigshotte, New Wokingham Road, Wokingham, Berks RG11 3AY

Colostomy Welfare Group, 38–39 Eccleston Square, London SW1V 1PB

Gamblers Anonymous, 17/23 Blantyre Street, London SW10

Ileostomy Association of Great Britain and Northern Ireland, 1st Floor, 23 Winchester Road, Basingstoke, Hants.

Mastectomy Association, 1 Colworth Road, Croydon, Surrey CR0 7AD

Migraine Trust, 45 Great Ormond Street, London WC1N 3AY

Multiple Sclerosis Society of Great Britain and Northern Ireland, 286 Munster Road, Fulham, London SW6 6AP

Psoriasis Association, 7 Milton Street, Northampton NN2 7JG

Royal National Institute for the Blind, 224 Great Portland Street, London W1N 6AA

Royal National Institute for the Deaf, 105 Gower Street, London WC1E 6AH

The Spastics Society, 12 Park Crescent, London W1N 4EQ